CARDIAC WELLNESS
HOW TO SUSTAIN THE LIFESTYLE CHANGES YOU NEED FOR A HEALTHY HEART

CARDIAC WELLNESS
HOW TO SUSTAIN THE LIFESTYLE CHANGES
YOU NEED FOR A HEALTHY HEART

LAWRENCE A. DECKER, PH.D.

Nova Science Publishers, Inc.
New York

This book is dedicated to my wife, Louise,
to my children, Elena and Jay,
to my sister Barbara,
and to the memory of my parents,
Dr. Robert J. Decker and Jeanette Estrin Decker

CONTENTS

ACKNOWLEDGEMENTS

This book would not have been possible without the help and support of many people.

If you find this book readable, it is because of my friend and editor, Hillary Lee. Her commitment to clarity, structure, excellence, and closure was a constant throughout the editing process. As an editor, she somehow combines the skills of a master psychologist, philosopher, teacher, and comedian.

My daughter, Elena, was a constant source of inspiration for me. She helped me to discover my own voice by demanding that I write letters about myself in a conversational tone. No one can turn a phrase or see things from a fresh perspective better than my artistic daughter.

As an active seventeen year old, my son Jay helps me to keep me fit and on my toes. I enjoy the time we spend together watching sporting events, and listening to his commentary and predictions. Jay doesn't pull any punches and, hopefully, that kind of directness has appeared in this book.

My sister and nephew Barbara and Matt Zerby were always there in the background egging me on to complete this work. Their gentle teasing and plain speaking influenced the tone of this book.

There are no better speakers for the real world than my friends Howard and Jill Savin. I cherish their critical insights. I could count on Howard and Jill to keep me grounded and realistic when I would lapse into wishful thinking.

Jeff and Andi Weiner were both instrumental in the writing of this book. These dear friends, by word and example, are all about possibility and creation. They encouraged me to "go for it" and never wavered from pushing me beyond my self imposed limits.

My friends, Dave and Patti Lieberman, helped me to structure my thoughts during long and enjoyable walks on the boardwalk. David helped me to transform my academic style of writing into colorful language and Patricia was a patient and attentive listener and advisor.

I give thanks to Doug & Susanne Sweeny and Jan & Jim Clayton for their support and guidance.

There were so many people who gave generously of their time to review this book and make comments that proved invaluable. John & Kathy Wallace, Shari & Ron Schiller, Kathy Ruth, David Clayton, Arnie Zeigel, Paul & Jackie Benner, Dave & Marti Goldthorpe, Gray Safford, Roland & Fran Bender, Brian & Caroline Horner, Ron Maltz, were just some of these people.

Jo-Lynne Worley was instrumental in guiding this book, particularly during the early stages of writing. Her keen insights were always welcome. Kathleen Lance and Lori Rea provided additional editing and direction.

I owe special gratitude to my patients, particularly the three core members of my heart group. My heart patients have taught me how to overcome obstacles by facing their demons. Their courage in the face of difficult circumstances gave me hope and inspiration. To the degree that you benefit from reading this book, it is because of their contributions.

On a more personal note, there is no way to categorize the contribution of my wife Louise. This is because she is part and parcel of who I have become. To the degree that I have developed emotional intelligence, it is because of her example. On a daily basis, she demonstrates integrity, empathy, and authenticity. These qualities show up in this book as steps towards heart health.

PREFACE

"If you look at people after coronary artery by-pass grafting two years later, 90% of them have not changed their lifestyle."
Dr. Edward Miller,
Dean of the Medical School at John Hopkins University

"What a fraud," I thought as I prepared to undergo another cardiac catheterization. For ten years I had been counseling heart patients at The Center for Cardiac Wellness, an institute which I had founded. Yet during this time my weight, my cholesterol, my triglycerides, and my blood pressure had all steadily risen. Worse still, my arteries were blocked again.

What had gone wrong? Why had I been unable to follow the advice that I gave to my clients? Why do relatively intelligent people like me, who have undergone a painful and life-threatening event such as coronary by-pass surgery, find they are facing additional painful procedures?

I am not the only one to ask these hard questions. Many patients with heart disease wonder why they can't seem to change their ways even when their lives are at stake. Dr. Edward Miller, Dean of the Medical School at John Hopkins University underscored the problem facing heart patients; only **one in ten** is successful in making necessary changes. He said, "If you look at people after coronary artery by-pass grafting, two years later, 90% of them have not changed their lifestyle." He went on to note that a significant number of angioplasties and by-pass operations require repeat procedures, suggesting that even in the face of life threatening disease, people don't seem to change their ways!

At-risk individuals who have not yet experienced symptoms of heart disease such as shortness of breath or angina or have not yet undergone risky surgical procedures may mistakenly assume that what hasn't happened won't happen. It is hard to give up unhealthy habits when they are associated with unimagined future events.

Open heart surgery is a risky and painful operation – one that should offer sufficient motivation to change your ways. Every day I wake up and am confronted by a thick 10 inch long scar in the center of my chest. Every night I take 4 different medications before going to bed. And every day I worry whether the various aches and pains I experience are signs that "the big one" is coming. You might think that these experiences would be incentive enough to adopt a healthy lifestyle. You would be wrong.

So why don't perfectly rational individuals follow their doctors' valuable recommendations? It turns out that the underlying factors derailing this good advice are energy and emotions. Heart patients are simply too exhausted and feel too depleted to sustain beneficial lifestyle choices. They *know* what they need to do and they *want* to comply, they just can't seem to consistently *act* on their good intentions.

Check out some of the staggering statistics associated with cardiovascular disease:

- almost two million Americans have a heart attack each year -- OVER A THIRD OF THEM DIE
- 43 % of Americans will die from some form of cardiovascular disease
- nation's number one killer of Americans over age 40
- 70 million Americans afflicted
- over one million people in the U.S. undergo invasive heart procedures each year (by-pass surgery, angioplasty)

The key to heart health lies in knowing:

> Heart Disease is essentially a disease of lifestyle.

Health professionals insist that lifestyle factors are as important in causing heart disease as traditional risk factors such as genetics, diabetes, high cholesterol, obesity, and hypertension. We know what lifestyle choices promote heart health. However, statistics prove that this knowledge alone is not enough to ensure that lifestyle changes will stick. The problem is the heart patients are too exhausted and depleted to follow through on what they know. Once you understand what's draining you and stem the outflow of energy, you're in a better position to stem the progression of coronary artery disease.

Dr. Dean Ornish of the Preventive Medicine Research Institute has shown that you can actually reverse the progression of coronary heart disease by sticking to a heart healthy lifestyle. By increasing your energy, you will be in a better position to exercise self control when you need it.

You probably have gathered loads of good ideas from the self help books out there. In fact, you probably know plenty about healthy choices for your ideal lifestyle. You can activate that valuable information and get the energy you need to put what you know into practice. This book tells you how. Finally, you will be able to effectively apply all of that positive information in a way that will make lasting changes.

AUTHOR'S NOTE

I wrote the book after coming to the humbling conclusion that there were unresolved issues outside my awareness that kept throwing me off track. Foremost was the discovery that I lacked emotional intelligence. I could not recognize and label many of my own feelings. Unable to manage my feelings effectively, I made choices that undermined my health.

In this book I have identified eight distinct obstacles. I will show you how to spot them and follow nine detailed steps to circumvent them. With the obstacles removed from your path, you will be on your way to sustaining a healthy lifestyle.

Obstacles to health are part of our prevailing culture. They stem from messages we have gotten all our lives, so they become like background noise to us. We come to accept these messages even though they undermine our well-being. The messages become beliefs which act as obstacles to our progress. Even though they are false beliefs, we accept them as true. This is especially evident with heart patients. We may not question our way of doing things until we are facing bright lights on the operating table. It takes energy to defend a position that is essentially untrue – energy that could be better used to sustain a healthy lifestyle.

Applying the principles in this book saved my life. These same principles extended the lives of my patients and can help you as well. My hope is that I will inspire you to become the *one in ten* I mention repeatedly in this book.

NOTE TO READER

Now is the time when your motivation for lifestyle change is the highest it will ever be.

If you have recently learned that you are at risk for heart disease or are about to undergo an invasive procedure, it would be useful to write down some of your thoughts and feelings about your heart disease, and save them in a journal. You want to pay particular attention to the battles you are engaged in on a day to day basis. These are the areas that are draining your energy. Pay attention to how frightened you might feel, how worried you are about your own capabilities in the future, your financial concerns, how your spouse and children will carry on as you recover, your capacity to do things around the house, and at work. Write about any misgivings you may have about how you treated your body, how you should have watched your weight, or had a few less beers, or exercised more. Write about any remorseful or guilty feelings you have. Write about your attempts to keep disturbing thoughts and feelings in check. Ask your spouse and kids to write a page in your journal about how they have felt during and after your procedure. What were their fears, concerns, issues?

Make a separate page for your resolutions. List the things you intend to do differently in the future, once you get on your feet. What kind of diet will you follow? How will you handle alcohol? What kind of exercise program will you start? How much time will you allocate to the kids, to vacation, to having fun with your spouse, to reading or smelling the roses?

I am asking you to do this now because there is a 90% chance that you will forget all that you wrote, and resume the same unhealthy lifestyle that contributed to your heart surgery. By having this journal written in your own words, you can periodically refer to it as a vivid reminder that you don't want to repeat this experience ever again. It will help increase the odds that you will stick to your resolutions. Reading and re-reading this book will strengthen your resolve as well.

Keep your journal with you as you read this book. It is important that you record any positive or negative experiences that come to mind as you read. At the end of each step, I will ask you three questions. You will get better results if you write your answers in your journal.

INTRODUCTION

WHAT WE'RE LOOKING AT

Heart patients are depleted and exhausted because they are doing battle on multiple fronts. In a very real way, they, face changes in their physical condition, their home and work life, leisure activities and so on. Internally, they must deal with toxic emotions such as anxiety, sadness, depression, fear, or anger. At the same time they are bombarded by unresolved issues of the past – childhood hurts that have not been adequately handled.

Heart patients are fighters. They try not to let disturbing thoughts and feelings into their lives. Over time, this suppression develops into a way of life – the Avoidant Lifestyle. So much energy is expended resisting painful realities that there is little energy left for curbing temptation or moving in a positive direction. This book seeks to help heart patients identify and deal with their stressors as well as their values. In doing so, energy is reclaimed that can be used for healthy living.

HOW THIS BOOK IS DIFFERENT

This book begins where most self-help books end. Most self help books prescribe behavior changes – better diet, more exercise – the same things you hear from your family and your doctors. They all urge you to make changes that will improve your health. You've probably followed some of that good advice for a while. But then you found yourself back with the same old unhealthy habits. No surprise. Your good ideas and your best intentions are sabotaged by factors outside your awareness. Your psychological defenses are draining you of the energy needed to make healthy lifestyle choices. This book will provide you with the tools to stop that energy drain and get back on track towards heart health. Only when you address the real reasons behind your inability to follow through on your good intentions can you become that *one in ten* who will stick to a heart-healthy plan.

This book addresses a baffling question: Why do perfectly sane people have lifestyles that are killing them? This book is designed to arm the reader with insight and ability to diagnose underlying emotional issues related to heart disease and to heal them. This strategy was developed by someone who is both a psychologist and a heart patient.

Cardiac Wellness provides a unique perspective on the relationship between Emotional Intelligence (the ability to recognize and regulate emotions) and heart disease. It offers a compelling theory linking psychological obstacles to heart disease, and details steps you can take to sustain a heart-healthy life.

Cardiac Wellness exposes a frightening reality: Your heart condition will probably worsen until you get a handle on your emotions. Remember, only *one in ten* people will adopt and sustain a heart-healthy lifestyle.

Get ready to change your life for good.

GETTING SET TO GO

**Only *one in ten* individuals with heart disease is successful in maintaining a heart healthy lifestyle.
Be that One.**

You are beginning a journey of inquiry – inquiry about areas related to your emotional well-being and heart health. This is uncharted territory. You don't know a lot about the places you will visit. By the end of your journey you will understand how each area you visited increases the odds that you can reverse heart disease.

Let's assume you know what you should be doing about your health. You've probably been hearing good advice from your doctor, your family, and everyone close to you. Increase your exercise, control your weight, relax, and stop smoking. You would think that the threat of illness or death would be sufficient motivation to follow their advice. Yet you can't seem to motivate yourself to follow through. In fact, you may be unmotivated to do much of anything beneficial. You're discouraged about your self-control and worried that your behavior is threatening your health. You are not alone. In fact, you are in the vast majority of heart patients.

Heart Disease is essentially a disease of lifestyle. The problem is, you don't have the energy to maintain a healthy lifestyle – to make good choices consistently. You *know* what you need to do and you *want* to comply but you just can't seem to consistently *act* on your good intentions. Whether you are aware of it or not, chances are that you are too exhausted and depleted to follow through on what you know. You start getting the behavior you really want only when you have energy available to make good decisions. Where do you get this energy?

The nature of your emotions powerfully influences the energy levels you experience. If you are angry, your body generates a pulse of energy strong enough for rage. If you are elated you can jump for joy. One action gets you in trouble; the other is its own reward. The more intense your emotional state, the more your energy level is affected. In order to conserve energy for the healthy activities you choose, you want to get a handle on your emotions. You want to increase your positive emotions and limit the toxic effects of your negative emotions.

> ## HANDLE YOUR EMOTIONS AND YOU WILL CHANGE YOUR RESULTS.

Consider what happens when you feel sad. You have little energy. It takes energy to exercise self-control. Without energy it is difficult to resist temptation. You engage in unhealthy behaviors and then think poorly of yourself. This makes you sadder.

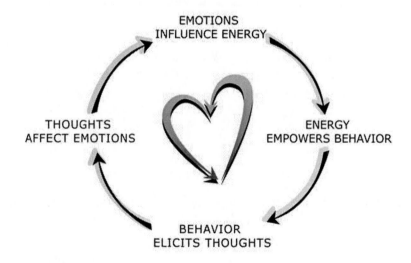

Figure I. Energy Cycle

Clearly, heart patients have less energy available because their hearts aren't working at 100% capacity. What is less well understood is that heart patients have less energy because they are busy defending themselves against emotional stress.

Heart patients are bombarded by external stressors – reduced physical capabilities, work issues, financial changes, etc. At the same time they are preyed on by internal stressors – worry about the future, anger or sadness about lost capabilities, loss of self-image, etc. Add to this toxic mix the unresolved emotional issues of the past and you have a stressed out heart patient with depleted reserves.

> THE KEY TO SUSTAINING A HEALTHY LIFESTYLE
> IS TO STEM THE OUTFLOW OF ENERGY BEING
> EXPENDED FOR DEFENSIVE PURPOSES.

What are "unresolved issues of the past"? We all suffered hurt feelings as children and many of us endured difficult times. These painful memories stay with us although they are usually below the surface. They resurface when a current circumstance reminds us of a similar circumstance in the past. For example, being faced with illness may rekindle old memories of being sick as a child. If you hated being treated like an invalid or were angry that you couldn't do things with your friends back then, the same kinds of feelings may come up for you in the present. These old feelings can be painful and add to the more obvious stressors associated with heart disease.

There is plenty of evidence that links adverse childhood experiences with unhealthy adult lifestyles and heart disease. According to Bessel van der Kolk, M.D. of Boston University Medical Center, "the more adverse childhood experiences a person reports, the more likely he or she is to develop life-threatening illnesses such as heart disease, and stroke." And C.L. Whitfield submitted an article which appeared in the 1998 American Journal of Preventive Medicine asserting that chronic disease "has its roots in unprocessed emotional experiences of childhood." The good news is: You don't have to go through lengthy psychotherapy to uproot these painful feelings. Just by acknowledging that they exist you can free up some of the energy that has been spent keeping these feelings from surfacing.

> ACKNOWLEDGING HURTFUL EXPERIENCES BEGINS
> UNLOCKING THEIR NEGATIVE POWER OVER YOU.

Excessive self control ultimately exhausts your supply of energy and leaves you vulnerable to temptation. Heart patients are exhausted because they attempt to control so much of their lives.

You can maintain and even increase your energy reserves by the following practices:

- CONJURE UP POWERFUL MEMORIES OF THE THINGS YOU VALUE IN LIFE -.Studies have shown that self-control is boosted when people recall memories of the things they value in life.

- FOCUS ON POSITIVE EMOTIONS – Love, laughter, and appreciation increases your energy while negative emotions like guilt and fear can deplete you.
- BECOME MORE AWARE OF YOUR EMOTIONS - You will have more energy available for self control by increasing your ability to recognize and handle your emotions.
- BE YOUR TRUE SELF - Energy is increased when you are being truly yourself. You have more energy because you are not pretending to be other than yourself and are not living in fear of being found out.
- FIND YOUR VOICE - When you learn to distinguish your own voice and recognize your intuition, you will have more energy to live a healthy life.
- LIVE IN THE MOMENT - When you live your life in the present moment there is more energy available to you for willpower and self control. This is because you are not letting your conditioned past run you nor are you postponing your life for some hoped for future event.
- LEARN TO ACCEPT WHAT IS SO - Accepting "what is" increases energy while resisting reality depletes energy. You can learn how to be more tolerant of even unpleasant realities. There is tremendous power in a shrug.
- IDENTIFY EXERCISE THAT APPEALS TO YOU – Make it fun; make it easy.
- MASTER SIMPLE TASKS – Small triumphs such as teaching yourself not to say "um" when you speak, will boost your energy reserves.

ACCEPTANCE VS. CONTROL

**You are never too far along the
wrong path to turn around.**

*Part of what you do in preparation for any journey is think about
what to take. What will the climate be? What will you need to
have on hand where you're going? There are things you will
need to bear in mind for this journey. Just for starters, accept
that you may be a little apprehensive of this journey.*

We all have internal experiences which we call thoughts or feelings. Maybe you
thought about telling your boss where to get off, or felt like passing that guy doing 25
in a 45 mile per hour zone. We are all challenged by our impulses. Give in to
temptation or resist? These questions assume that we are aware of our thoughts or
feelings – aware enough to make a decision. At a deeper level, we can ask the
question "Do I accept my thoughts or feelings as I experience them, or seek to control
my internal experiences?"

Many heart patients are unaware of their internal experiences – they are too busy
dealing with "important" issues. It takes energy to govern your internal experiences –
energy to regulate or control what you think or feel. The human body uses energy to
fuel all its activities. Self control is one such activity. Without energy you cannot
exert self control or willpower.

Research conducted by Roy Baumeister of Florida State University demonstrated
that a person is less able to resist temptations once self control is exercised in another
area. If you exert energy managing your impression on other people you will be less

likely to resist those potato chips. In order to get around this problem, you will need to be very selective about how you spend your energy.

To exercise self control means that you regulate your thoughts or feelings. You often do this in order to make healthy choices. For example, when you choose to exercise despite an urge to sleep in, or skip the donut despite the temptation to swallow it whole, you are exercising self control. Sometimes you can have too much of a good thing, however.

There are times when governing your thoughts or feelings is not healthy. When you habitually override, resist, restrain, constrict, suppress, or regulate your internal experiences, you are saying to yourself, "My experience is not ok as it is. I can't deal with this." It is this lack of acceptance of your thoughts and feelings that costs you energy. Of course we can't live in society without exercising self control. How many marriages would survive if you answered honestly the question "Do I look good in this?" Mental control can be a significant energy drain. It costs you extra to alter your experiences.

Keeping your feelings in check or trying to stop yourself from thinking certain thoughts are forms of altering your experience. Many heart patients experienced emotional wounding as children. They learned early in life to think or say words to this effect; "It's not alright with me. It shouldn't be this way". As adults, they are primed to react the same way when faced with painful circumstances.

For heart patients, saying "no" to our experiences is a common occurrence. When it comes to trusting others, experiencing our emotions, expressing ourselves or even being ourselves, we may have learned to be very cautious. These defensive operations leave less energy for other important areas of life, such as pursuing goals, living up to ideals with respect to health, spirituality or community life, and realizing our virtues as a spouse, parent, or friend.

It may be very true that the conditions we faced as children were harsh and intolerable. But in order to deal with any problem, you must first acknowledge it.

> THE KEY TO BEING MAKING PEACE WITH OUR PAST
> IS BEING ABLE TO REVIEW OUR EXPERIENCES
> WITHOUT NEEDING TO ALTER THEM.

WHAT NEEDS TO BE ACCEPTED?

Acceptance does not mean that you like the situation you are in. Nor does it imply putting up with negative situations. Of course you should get out of an abusive relationship or a disastrous job. Acceptance is a way of considering thoughts and feelings in a new light. When you simply observe uncomfortable thoughts and painful feelings in a detached way, you reduce their harmful effect on you. By your willingness to look with detachment upon the situations in your life, you diminish their power over you. You have more control because you are choosing to allow something into your awareness.

EMOTION-AVOIDANCE CYCLE OF DISEASE

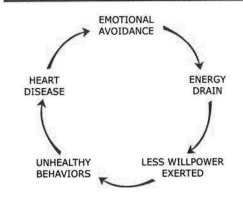

EMOTION-ACCEPTANCE CYCLE OF HEALTH

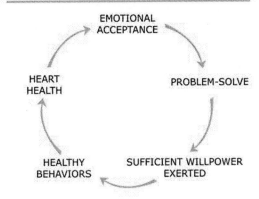

Figure II. Health / Disease Cycle

Acceptance means that even your unpleasant memories and sensations are acknowledged rather than suppressed. Studies have shown that people who are willing to re-experience the memories, thoughts and feelings that child abuse produces are less affected by the abuse. People who cannot make room for their distressing feelings have a very hard time with self control. For example, if you are unwilling to experience anxiety you are likely to feel far more anxiety--even panic. Remember, you are not being asked to approve of any aspect of your experience. You are asked simply to be a detached observer for yourself. The payoff is significant: By allowing your experiences to be reviewed you are gaining energy. Acceptance is the cornerstone of health.

Breaking Out of the Cycle

> *For most destinations there is a guidebook. For this journey, all the information you need is contained within you.*

Looking back on my 35 years as a Clinical Psychologist, I have treated hundreds of patients for symptoms relating to lifestyle. My patients engaged in overeating, problem drinking, smoking, sedentary habits, and drug abuse as a response to specific stressful life circumstances – vain attempts to cope with painful feelings. I discovered two disturbing facts about lifestyle and chronic disease. First, unhealthy behavior patterns contributed to the onset of patients' disease conditions, and second, after being diagnosed with a chronic disease, unhealthy behaviors continued to negatively affect the course of their disease. When it comes to cardiac diseases, compliance with doctor recommendations for improving lifestyle is often a matter of life or death. Yet the record shows that these patients are highly resistant to lifestyle changes.

This is not mere theory for me. I have struggled with lifestyle issues my entire life. It was a losing battle, resulting in quadruple coronary by-pass surgery. It took years of unhealthy living to clog my arteries. Even after surgery it took years to figure out what I was doing wrong. Just as you undoubtedly do, I knew what to do; I just couldn't seem to get myself to do it. It turned out that the factors that kept me from sustaining a healthy lifestyle had a lot to do with fighting too many battles at once. My willpower was being depleted by constantly putting out fires. I've got news for you that will probably come as a great relief: You can learn what makes you tick and use it to get on track and stay on track. The key is in understanding and working with—not against—yourself.

Working against yourself results in a vicious cycle of discouragement in which your family members watch helplessly as your condition deteriorates. Frustrated by ineffectiveness, family members may accuse you of lacking self-discipline, further depleting your self esteem. You get more depressed and end up back in the cardiologist's office with additional problems. And it continues until you: BREAK OUT OF THE CYCLE.

At some point each and every high risk individual has to ask, "Am I going to continue along a slow path to destruction, or am I going to recognize what's killing me and do something about it?"

DOING SOMETHING ABOUT IT

What kind of heart patient increases the odds of survival? In other words, who is the *one in ten* that sustains the lifestyle changes necessary for his survival?

One in ten has learned to open his heart emotionally, so that he is not at the effect of painful buried memories. He recognizes and handles arrogance and envy, as these states arise. He listens to others and to himself, instead of listening for confirmation of his point of view. He is aware of his defensiveness as it shows up in his thinking and influences his behavior. He has learned to identify his emotions and can express what he is feeling in ways that maximize his chances of being heard. He is present to the experiences of the moment. He has developed the capacity to put himself in others' shoes. He has become less preoccupied with himself, and more concerned about others. He is comfortable with his place in the world, and takes pleasure in other's success and happiness. He is genuinely appreciative of those people who offer help to him, and has learned to let love into his life. He is less subject to emotional hijacking because he is aware of what triggers him. He has reduced the impact of painful memories by talking about them with people he trusts. He has more energy for self control because he has stopped suppressing so many of his experiences. He no longer defines himself as a limiting set of beliefs formed in childhood, but now sees himself as someone who shapes, molds, and chooses who he is and how he lives.

"Sound's wonderful!" you say. "How do I get from here to there?"

JOURNEY TO A HEALTHY LIFE

The journey of a thousand miles begins with a single step. Along the way you will encounter obstacles. You'll be expecting them and you'll be able to go around them when they show up. You'll be directed through a series of nine steps. Some will require soul-searching; others will bring you unanticipated relief from emotional pain. Following these steps will lead you to the emotional health necessary to support a heart healthy lifestyle. What you discover about yourself along the way will transform you. The authentic you that will emerge during your journey will be fully capable of designing and maintaining a lifestyle consistent with your renewed commitment to your well being.

JOURNAL REFLECTION

Do you engage in unhealthy behaviors when your willpower is low? What behaviors?

OBSTACLES

The least initial deviation from the truth is multiplied later a thousandfold.
Aristotle

> *All journeys have their pitfalls. Read up on the obstacles you are likely to encounter along the way. Recognize them and go around them.*

Obstacles to health are part of our prevailing culture. They stem from messages we have gotten all our lives so they become like background noise to us. We come to accept these messages even though they undermine our well-being. They are essentially "no" messages rather than "yes" messages; they are constrictive rather than expansive. They undermine our well-being because they narrow our lives rather than open our lives to new experiences.

These early messages become beliefs which act as obstacles to our progress. Even though they are false beliefs, we accept them as true. This is especially evident with heart patients. We may not question our way of doing things until we are in a crisis situation. It takes energy to defend a position that is essentially untrue – energy that could be better used to sustain a healthy lifestyle.

There are eight fundamental obstacles along the path to emotional soundness. Examine these false notions:

1. Keep Your Guard Up

Heart patients don't want to be vulnerable. They develop strategies to protect themselves. When you keep your guard up you can't let in the love you need. The message you hear is "Don't trust".

2. Put On a Happy Face
Feelings of shame and experiences of invalidation lurk in the minds of many heart patients. Emotional trauma cannot be overcome by simple edicts such as "snap out of it" or "cheer up". Ignoring emotional pain only prolongs and intensifies it. When it comes to painful experiences, the message you may hear is "Don't Feel".

3. We Are Our Genes
More and more research indicates that social and emotional factors play a significant part in the development of heart disease – that they are on par with traditional risk factors such as family history. It is not true that "This can't be helped." You can overcome the edict "Don't act" when you understand that you do have control of your health.

4. Keep Up With the Joneses
Advertising and business interests bombard you with the myth that material possessions will bring you satisfaction. What you have is not good enough, not sufficient. Materialism appeals to people who feel empty or one down. When you can't appreciate what you already have, "Don't be content" is the message you hear.

5. Bite Your Tongue
Toxic feelings often lie buried in the wake of painful experiences. Toxic waste can prevent us from getting the love we need and living the life of our dreams. We need to express our painful feelings, not just bite our tongues. "Don't express" is the message to overcome.

6. Logic Saves the Day
Heart patients want to be in control, to be reasonable, but reactions aren't always governed by logic. Emotions cannot simply be ignored. There needs to be a balance between emotions and reason. The message "Don't be emotional" must be challenged.

7. What's Done Is Done
People are neurologically wired in such a way that memories of early trauma are triggered over and over again – until they learn to deal with them. It is hard to experience peace when the unwelcome memories keep surfacing. "Don't remember" is the message to overcome.

8. Keep Your Act Together
Heart patients often wear masks while living out their lives. They show themselves to be tough and in control, or kind and caring, all the while covering feelings of shame and inadequacy. In order to live authentically, they must resolve these feelings and remove their masks. The message to overcome is "Don't reveal".

JOURNAL REFLECTION

Do you take issue with labeling any of the above as "obstacles"? If so, which ones seem to be useful guidelines to you? Explain.

STEPS TO A HEART HEALTHY LIFESTYLE

Give me health and a day and I will make the pomp of emperors ridiculous.
Emerson

To get where you want to go efficiently, follow a well-marked map.

Just as there are obstacles to avoid on your path, there are key steps to take. The obstacles sap your energy whereas these steps re-energize you. Remember that obstacles are "no" messages—messages that say "Don't go there". In contrast, these steps are "yes" messages—messages that open your heart. Taken with confidence, they will alter your life for good.

THE 9 STEPS TO EMOTIONAL HEALTH

STEP 1)-Open Your Mind

To be truly open to new ideas requires that you trust yourself and others. You can review the basic principles and beliefs which you have taken for granted without fear. This is a key step toward emotional soundness.

STEP 2)-Tune in

In order to discover your authentic self, you must first resolve the dialogue in your head. Recognizing your defensive voice is vital to emotional awareness.

STEP 3)-Take Responsibility

Begin to see how you were instrumental in bringing about the situations in your life and that you have a say in how things turn out. Responsibility is the backdrop to all health.

STEP 4)-Acceptance Begins the Process of Healing

Acceptance of those painful things from your past that you cannot change sets the stage for healing. You get to appreciation through acceptance.

STEP 5)-Cleanse your mind

Letting go of harmful emotions increases your peace of mind and frees you from reacting to the least provocation.

STEP 6)-Act with Integrity

In order to make wise decisions and act with integrity, you must be present and aware. You must have access to your thoughts, feelings and values.

STEP 7)-Live in the Moment

You need to be present in order to recharge your batteries. Living in the past or waiting for the future is draining.

STEP 8)-Let Love In

Intimacy is like salve to an open wound. You need to be yourself in order for love to heal and empower you.

STEP 9)-Create a New Mission

Recognize your dearest desires and design the rest of your life from inside out – from your heart to the rest of the world.

From this point on you move forward with new awareness. It is the beginning of your conscious chosen life. Now comes the moment of true creation. You discover that you have transformed yourself. Your life is no longer about doing or having in an endless quest for future security. Your life is about living in the moment and being yourself. You no longer hide behind your lifestyle, soothing yourself with short term fixes that destroy your vitality. You no longer identify yourself with your limited beliefs, your story, or your unhealthy lifestyle. You are free to choose your life and create yourself anew at every moment.

"Many people can begin to reverse their heart disease simply by changing their lifestyle."

Dr. Dean Ornish
Director of the Preventive Medicine Research Institute

THE JOURNEY BEGINS

Step 1 – Open Your Mind

Are you eager and excited? – nervous? Be bold; begin the journey.

Open Your Mind to the possibility that there is a better way for you to live your life.

We all want to think we are open to new ideas. In truth, we are accepting ideas that already fit with our notions of "reality". Really new ideas are disturbing to most people because they threaten to rock the boat. You've heard about the reaction Galileo got when he proposed the outrageous idea that the earth actually circles around the sun.

To be really open to new ideas means that the basic principles and beliefs that you have taken for granted are up for review. Even the very foundations on which you have based your life may be disputed.

It's hard to be open. It is human nature to avoid rocking the boat for fear of falling out. We choose the devil we know. Even our nervous systems are wired for familiarity and routine. We can get pretty worked up over things that seem unusual or out of place. Humans and animals alike seem to acclimate to circumstances – even noxious circumstances. We put up with polluted air, poverty, and even abuse, as long as those circumstances develop gradually. We are addicted to being right. It is almost as if we would rather be right than happy, or even alive. If you have chosen a particular path in life, or hold a particular belief dearly, you will be reluctant to give up that belief. We will wage wars to defend the "rightness" of our beliefs.

How can you be more open? Simply by recognizing that you may be resistant to new ideas you expand your openness. Many people go through their lives with rigid beliefs about how things should be done. They have no clue about the possibility of seeing things from other points of view. This may have characterized how you used to be. However, the fact that you are reading this suggests that you are open to considering new ways of looking at things. Your willingness is part of the first step to heart health.

MY PERSONAL STEP 1

I come from a background where there was a lot of family insecurity. We were financially strapped, without a father for long periods of time, and always anxious about his medical condition.

My comfort comes, in part, from familiarity. Even my dog becomes hysterical whenever the wind blows or an unfamiliar sound is heard. I am drawn to establishing routines.

I have to make the same conscious effort that you do when I am confronted with new ways of thinking that challenge my beliefs. But, because I've experienced the liberating payoff, I am willing to rethink and consider even controversial ideas.

I had all kinds of great ideas about how I was going to get back to health. For example, I reasoned that if I learned to think of myself as a worthwhile and deserving person, I would somehow treat my body with more respect, eat right and exercise properly. Further, I thought that by educating myself about the risk factors of heart disease and the proper behaviors to reduce risk that I would straighten myself out. I was fooling myself.

I had no idea how hard it would be to accomplish these goals. I made every mistake in this book: I kept thinking that I could stick to a healthy lifestyle by just making up my mind; I could do this by myself without asking for help; I already knew all about myself so there was nothing new to learn; I was smarter than most people so I could use reason to stay on track.; my lapses into unhealthy behaviors were not my fault; I would get my life together some time in the future; I was perfectly content to be alone so it didn't matter if I kept disappointing my family; I was already in a helping profession so I really didn't need to focus on anyone other than myself.

My mistake was that I didn't know enough about myself. You can't see the truth if you are blind. I didn't realize that my good intentions could be so easily sabotaged by emotional factors. As a psychologist, I thought I was immune to fooling myself. After all, I knew all about defenses – could identify them easily in my patients. I could spot when someone *else* was in denial; I could spot rationalization from a hundred paces – *in others*. And I knew all about distraction. You couldn't fool me. It was a rude awakening to discover that I too had blind spots.

While open heart surgery paved the way for my recovery from blocked arteries, my doctor could only do so much. He gave me the chance to live, but could do nothing to ensure that I would take advantage of the opportunity. And, like me, he did not totally understand how difficult it would be to change my life habits.

I learned that the opening of my emotional heart was necessary to increase the odds that the heart surgeon's good works were not wasted. By opening up the emotional heart, I do not mean becoming more loving and expressive of warm and tender feelings (although that certainly is a desired outcome). What I found even more difficult, but necessary, was uncovering the painful feelings that held me hostage to self protective and self defeating behaviors. I had to become more open to my experiences, and more willing to consider my heart disease in a whole new light.

OBSTACLE 1: KEEP YOUR GUARD UP

> *You're opening your mind and starting to feel vulnerable. It's tempting to try and get away from this uncomfortable feeling, to rationalize it away. When your mind throws out this reservation as you take that first step, you are encountering the first obstacle. Don't panic. You were expecting obstacles along the way, right? Let's examine this one more closely:*

Experience can be the best teacher if we are open to it. But if you keep having the same experience over and over again, there is not much learning possible. Heart patients are not often trusting. They don't want to be vulnerable; they won't risk being hurt…again. They develop strategies to protect themselves. When you keep your guard up you can't be open to new experiences.

DEFENSE MECHANISMS

One reason why we can't think our way unerringly through life is that our ability to see accurately is clouded by filters – our defense mechanisms. These are like sentinels guarding against our perceiving things as they really are. Their job is to alter the way we assess reality so that we don't suffer from it. Our defense mechanisms cause us to make assessments about risk that are based more upon our wishes than upon reality. For example, people erroneously estimate the probability of death from heart disease to be about a third less than actual statistics indicate.

Many heart patients so overuse their defense mechanisms that they don't learn from their experiences. Once they make up their minds, new information can't get through. For example, you meet a new person named Jane. You think that Jane is "just like" Mary. If that is true for you, it is difficult to see Mary as a new person.

Bill, 90 years old and on his deathbed says, "Son, I knew what's so when I was 4 years old and I haven't changed my mind since." Guess what Bill has been doing for 86 years!

Psychological defenses operate unconsciously. Defense mechanisms, established to make us feel better, can end up taking over our lives. If we suffered repeated emotional wounding as children, our defenses helped us to minimize the hurtful feelings that resulted from our negative experiences. Over-reliance on psychological defenses however, plays havoc with reality and destroys our lives.

When we are defensive, we are saying "No" to our present moments, robbing ourselves of our experiences. We are substituting some washed out, watered down, clouded over version of reality for the real thing because we haven't yet learned how to identify and handle our feelings.

DENIAL

Denial is simply wishful thinking: "Go ahead, have that dessert. One day of splurging is not going to affect your heart." You use this defense mechanism to lessen your anxiety about doing something that you know is unhealthy for you. This is a distortion or falsification of reality. But a part of you doesn't care. "It's a small price to pay to make me feel better." Or you tell yourself it's OK to go back to work after a heart attack without planning a realistic program of rehabilitation. This is wishful thinking that can kill you.

REPRESSION

Repression is the most powerful defense. If reality is simply too painful to endure, you will bury the thoughts, feelings and memories associated with the pain. You may have forgotten how depressed, fearful or angry you were as a child when you were mistreated or invalidated. Those memories have been repressed. You repress painful experiences because you intend for them to stay away. The problem is, they don't stay away. In fact, these memories are often easily triggered, requiring you to remain on guard.

LISTENING "FOR" VS. LISTENING "TO"

There are other ways in which we filter reality. Take everyday listening for example. Listening is different from hearing. If our ears operate normally, we can hear another's communication, but we may not process what is said (listen) correctly. We may not be listening to hear the message; we may be listening "for" something. The problem with listening "for" is that you've already made up your mind.

For example, my wife asks me a simple question, "Did you take your medication?" If, for a change, I listen to her question (without running it through a gauntlet of possible meanings), I might respond simply with a yes or no. It wouldn't be beyond me to misread her question and take it to be a subtle form of criticism. In my mind, I might hear her say, "I'm tired of looking after you like a two year old. When are you going to take responsibility for your own health and take your medicine without my having to remind you?" It is my interpretation of her question that will determine whether I look for my bottle of medicine or an argument.

Other times I presume to know ahead of time what she "really" means by her communication. "Obviously, she thinks I'm too stupid to remember my medication," I might think. Even though this might be far from the truth, I am listening "for" signs that she is being critical of me, instead of listing "to" what she has to say. Most of us are listening "for" something instead of "to" someone.

Things you listen "for" point to your areas of sensitivity – things that might pose a threat to you. You have defenses which work like radar, screening the airwaves for recognizable patterns to protect you against attack. Attacks may be perceived in simple gestures: She raised her eyebrow. "Now I know for sure she thinks I'm stupid."

When you catch yourself listening "for" something, you can bet you're not giving your full attention "to" what is being said. Listening "for" something is a signal that you are being defensive. You are preparing for battle just in case what you are looking for does or doesn't appear on your radar screen. You are on alert. Fight or flight hormones are coursing through your body. And nothing has happened yet! Listening "for" robs you of energy that could have been used more productively elsewhere – like exercising willpower.

When you listen for signs of approval or respect, you are anxious or worried about what others think of you. Whether or not signs of approval or respect show up on your radar screen, damage has already occurred because anxiety and worry have moved into your mind.

Think of the stress you subject yourself to by continuously scanning the airwaves for possible threat! If you habitually look "for" signs that people are out to con you, take advantage of you, make you look foolish, use you, or put you down, it is no wonder you feel "sick and tired" of how you are being treated.

It doesn't have to be this way. Once you recognize that a part of you is listening "for" something, you can identify what it is that you are listening "for." Then listen to what is being said. If you are really ambitious, you can try to figure out *why* you are listening for whatever it is you listen for. Chances are that an insecure self image is involved.

JOURNAL REFLECTION – STEP 1

When you start a new journey, are you more excited or worried?
Is it painful to remember much about your childhood? Why?
What do you listen "for"?

STEP 2 – TUNE IN

> *Simply becoming aware that your defense mechanisms are keeping you from seeing reality clearly is great progress – your mind is definitely opening! Now that you are aware you've been screening what gets into your conscious mind, you've successfully maneuvered around a significant obstacle. Carry on and learn what else is going on inside your mind.*

Learn to identify your inner voices to discern helpful guidance.

We all play many roles and wear many disguises. We want to make a good impression, to please our audience. These facades, our false fronts, are designed to mask a person we fear to reveal – the real us. Your acting is directed and coached by a dialog that takes place in your head. In order to discover your authentic self, you must first evaluate the dialogue in your head.

"What dialog?" you say. You know the one, that inner chatter that is never silent, that constantly argues with itself: "Go, ahead, have ice cream on top of your cake!" only to counter with "No, you can't afford the calories." Your inner voices are like characters vying for your attention. Ultimately, you will obey the most convincing one. These characters are positively ingenious at presenting you with compelling reasons why you should take their advice.

One voice speaks to you from a position of entitlement. This "royal voice" points out, "You deserve a drink after all you've gone through!" It employs your past conditioning and defense mechanisms to get you to ignore painful realities. When you hear yourself saying "should" a lot, there is a good chance that your arrogant royal voice is talking through you.

Jack Trimpey, author of *Rational Recovery--the New Cure for Substance Addiction* describes the "addictive voice". Recognizing this voice is a method for controlling substance abuse. Yet another voice talks to you about taking care of your health. This is your "voice of reason." When you can hear this voice above the chatter, you are getting wise counsel.

Your voices use a variety of pronouns: "I don't need to take my medication this morning." "You can skip one day's dosage without doing any harm." "Let's skip your medication today and sleep in." You can learn to catch a defensive voice talking because it is telling you to do something that is not in your long term best interest.

It is important to keep in mind that you are not your internal voices. You are the one giving rise to your internal voices. For the heart patient, these voices usually appear in one of two guises. One royal voice can appear arrogant while the other can appear to be quite humble. Though they will continue to vie for your attention, once you learn to recognize them for the characters they are, you will have taken the second step.

MY PERSONAL STEP 2

After one of my seminars, a client, Lloyd, approached me and enthusiastically declared that he had heard an internal conversation (with himself) for the first time in his life. Lloyd was over 70 years old! I asked myself, "How could he not be familiar with his own inner conversations? Could he really spend an entire life oblivious to the fact that entire conversations were going on in his head?"

In my opinion, the reason that Lloyd did not hear internal conversations was that the royal voice drowned out his own voice. Lloyd was extremely defensive. His inner life was taken over by the "King." He saw the world through the king's eyes and never questioned the king's observations or the king's authority. He obeyed without question and never heard his own voice in protest. There was no conversation going on in Lloyd's head; only the king's monologue.

By the way, Lloyd represents the kind of king I refer to as the "humble" type. He appears shy and quiet on the surface, a follower of protocol and proponent of social graces. Everyone likes Lloyd and in fact, he is a very giving person. You have to scratch beneath the surface to see the rebellious spirit, the stubborn, ambitious and arrogant person who has lived life on his own terms.

I believe that the humble king, in contrast to the overtly arrogant and visibly commanding king, is more defensive and less able to hear his own voice, than the openly arrogant king. Perhaps Lloyd was subjected to more subtle forms of invalidation as a child than the king who becomes visibly arrogant.

Lloyd's inner voice will caution against direct assaults. He is likely to mislabel his arrogant behaviors as being "helpful" or may see himself as "simply" being clear about what he wants instead of being dominating.

The type of king (or queen) I have referred to as arrogant will speak in an angry and defiant voice: "screw it, just do it!" or "I want it – end of story." You know where you stand when an arrogant king speaks his mind. When you hear yourself telling everyone in sight how things "should" be done there is a good chance that your arrogant king or queen is talking through you.

"People should behave towards me with reverence and respect, as if I were royalty," I might think. Or, "He should do this," and "They should do that." Of course, when the world didn't do what it "should," as demanded by the king or queen's mouthpiece (me), I would get angry. As you can imagine, I was angry a lot. Once I got off my high horse, and refused to listen to the king's demands I was able to be more accepting of others, just the way they are.

———————

It can be very entertaining, not to mention enlightening, to eavesdrop. One day I was listening in on my internal chatter. I wasn't feeling well; I was feeling depleted and worthless. I saw an ad in the paper for a spiffy new car. My conversation went something like this:

ROYAL VOICE: "Look at that car. I want it. I would get more respect from people if I pulled up in a car like that. I wouldn't feel like such a loser."

VOICE OF REASON: "I don't think having a spiffy car would do much to make me feel better. Besides, if I bought it I'd be saddled with debt".

ROYAL VOICE: "You deserve a car like that. You have done without for long enough. If you pay it off over five years, you wouldn't miss the money each month. Besides, your wife would be so proud of you when you go somewhere. Why don't we buy it?"

VOICE OF REASON: "I don't know."

ROYAL VOICE: "If your wife resists, you have every right to get angry. Look what you've done for her. She should do this for you without question."

You're beginning to get that the chatter never ends – you just get better at hearing your wisdom over the distracting din of the other voices.

———————

*For the story of how I discovered my inner voice (His Majesty, King Larry) see Appendix B.

OBSTACLE 2: PUT ON A HAPPY FACE

Can you believe how much conversation is going on inside your mind!? Did you catch any of the characters vying for your attention during that last step? Wait a minute…what is that looming up ahead? Not another obstacle!

You can do it. Remember how successfully you navigated around the last one? You know, the obstacle that kept you thinking in the same old way. This one should be quite familiar once you get up close to it.

Feelings of shame and experiences of emotional wounding are in the background of many heart patients. We see that emotional trauma cannot be overcome simply tuning out. Following edicts such as "snap out of it" or "cheer up" only mask the pain.

We are sometimes taught by our parents to smile through our pain, as if this will make our pain easier to bear. Inadvertently, by trying to help in this fashion, the parent invalidates the child.

Parent:	"How was school today?"
Child:	"Billy started calling me names again, so I decked him."
Parent:	"You *what!*?"
Child:	(crying) "But all the kids are calling me names now."
Parent:	"Just remember, you can attract more bees with honey."
Child:	"Huh?"

The child was cut to the core by the teasing, yet his feelings were invalidated by the parent's response. Invalidation results whenever feelings are punished, trivialized, disregarded, mislabeled or dismissed. A steady diet of invalidation will lead a child to protect himself from emotional wounding. Ultimately he may stop trusting others. He may learn to keep his feelings to himself. He can even train himself not to feel anything at all.

One day I was upset because I couldn't invite a friend over. Rather than attempt to understand or soothe my sad feelings, my father said, "If you keep it up, I'll give you something to really cry about." In this case, my experience of painful emotions was disregarded, and I felt threatened to boot. My father also used to tell me that I was "lazy" when in fact I was fearful or anxious about doing something for the first time. I was afraid I might fail. Since my father would occasionally add that he felt "manipulated" by my behavior, I became confused regarding my intentions and motivations. "Don't feel" was the message I ultimately obeyed.

Invalidation can come in several forms, as you will see in the case histories presented in this book. One of my patients, Arthur, was wounded by parents who did not recognize him as an individual. Mary was hurt by parents who could not demonstrate their love unconditionally. Sam was invalidated by parents who could not consider any of his desires legitimate, and Bernie was damaged by overprotective parents.

I was leading a group of heart patients, and asked them to write about their traumatic experiences, experiences that they thought may have influenced how their lives turned out. What these stories have in common is some kind of emotional trauma. Following is a sampling:

- ♥ I was 4 year old. My father hated immigrants. My best friend, an immigrant, came over to play with her new kitten. My father flew into a rage, and threw the kitten in the sky and killed it. My friend and I both screamed. I was sent to my bedroom and told to keep my hands folded. Looking at my father's violence, I made up my mind then and there to never get married and I didn't.

- ♥ I was almost 2 years old. We were at a picnic and my sister looked like she was crawling towards the water. I thought she could drown. I screamed for help. My parents came running. They laughed at me. I felt like a window came down. I said to myself, "How can you laugh when I am crying". I learned to keep my feelings to myself.

- ♥ I was about 4 years old. My father was leaving on a train for war. Everyone was crying and I was frightened. He was killed when I was 5. My mother was devastated. She became very close to me. But then she remarried and I felt abandoned by her. Then I became close to my grandmother, but my mother felt she was spoiling me, and we moved away. I had overwhelming sadness and was terrified of losing my grandmother. My mother did not allow me to cry and I was afraid of her. I doubted my courage and felt like a "sissy". Later I became a cop. It helped me hide my feelings of being a coward.

♥ My dad died when I was 2. My mom remarried a jerk, who used to hit me and call me a girl. As a guy, I was humiliated. I carried this with me all my life, afraid that people would think I was weak or feminine. I don't feel like a regular human being, and could never get close to people, or feel like I fit in. I became a public servant later and I tried to fit in, but always kept my distance.

♥ My own father took sick in the Navy and spent years in and out of hospitals. I remember him screaming out for morphine, when I was about 3 or 4. When he was home, he was very harsh with me. I was scared of him. My mother had to take over his magazine sales business to support the family. I was ashamed of my family life. I was alone a lot, and we had no money. My sister was born when I was 5, and she just added to the chaos. I am still afraid of abandonment and over react to conflict. I became a psychologist probably to figure myself out.

What these stories have in common is some kind of emotional trauma. Emotional trauma can be defined as the experiencing of an "Invalidating Environment" repeatedly. An invalidating environment is one in which the communication of feelings is met by erratic, or extreme responses. In other words, the expression of private experiences is not validated. Instead, the feelings that are shared are often punished, trivialized, disregarded, mislabeled or dismissed.

It is important to point out that the parents or caretakers who may have hurt the child's feelings, may not have been bad people. They did the best that they could do with the cards that they were dealt. Many were dealt a tough hand. My father was chronically ill and almost died. My mother had to support the family. What damage was done to me was incidental to their attempts to survive a tough set of circumstances.

It is hard to underestimate the damage that is inflicted when your private experiences are invalidated. What happens over time is that you learn to distrust your inner experiences, indeed become blind to them. You lose the ability to identify your own emotions. You can even lose the ability to feel loved. Genuine self love is impossible when your own experiences are unwelcome.

People who have been repeatedly wounded as children, learn to look at their own experiences with a jaundiced eye – they attempt to get away from their feelings. Instead of recognizing and dealing with their emotions, which would enable them to grow stronger, they have a few drinks, go to the gym, watch television, or work long hours – all in the service of distancing themselves from their "unacceptable" experiences.

Heart patients are not the only people on the planet who have suffered from difficult circumstances growing up. I think what sets heart patients apart from others (aside from their genetic makeup), is the extent to which heart patients have internalized, or taken to heart the invalidating experiences of childhood. Perhaps heart patients have experienced emotional wounding more frequently or more intensely than others. Or perhaps heart patients are born with more sensitivity than others. In any case, for a child, the physiological cost of repeated invalidation is heightened vigilance, more sensitivity to threat, and a depleted set of reserves.

An adult with depleted reserves is in a precarious position. The slightest threat could put him over the edge. He would see threat behind every tree and under every rock. Exhausted from being always on edge, his willpower would be depleted, leaving him more likely to engage in risky behaviors. He would also be exquisitely sensitive to anything remotely resembling a put down or a slight.

I am often sensitive to the point of absurdity. As embarrassing as it is for me to admit, I often find the need to "correct" my wife if she fails to include me in her conversation. She might say, "I had a great time at the zoo" – an appropriate response to a question addressed directly to her about how she spent her day. Somehow, I find it necessary to interject that I was there too. My heightened sensitivity to invalidation or rejection can lead me to see a slight where none was intended and to push for recognition inappropriately.

It gets even worse. If truth be told, I am even envious of my two dogs. They seem to get unconditional positive regard, stroking, and feeding from my wife.

Even today, I am taken aback when I am told that my problems sustaining lifestyle changes are due to "laziness." Many well meaning people don't understand that failing to sustain necessary lifestyle changes is a problem that can't be moralized out of existence. If it were simply a question of mind over matter, the odds wouldn't be so stacked against us.

SHAME

Shame is perhaps the most painful emotion we have. No one talks about their shame. When you feel ashamed of yourself, you want to curl up in a ball and hide. Nothing is as invalidating as shame. Shame is as close to self-hate as a person can come. When we are ashamed, we think that no one could possibly love us or even want to be with us. It is worse than guilt. You feel guilty when you do something that violates your standards. But when you feel ashamed, your very core of being is damaged. It's not what you do that's the problem; it's who you are that's at fault. Certain people can feel so ashamed of themselves that they would rather die than expose their perceived shortcomings. It would be a rare occurrence when I would admit that I was wrong about something. To do so could expose my ignorance, and bring up shameful memories of being called "stupid" by my father.

In order to avoid feelings of shame I have learned that the best defense is a good offense. By appearing to be arrogant and contemptuous and by one-upping everyone in sight, I can hide my fear of being seen as flawed, inadequate, unworthy and unlovable. Many of my heart patients are also masters at hiding their shame behind a wall of arrogance. My more humble heart patients may hide these same feelings by seeking to please others – often at their own expense.

When you grow up feeling ashamed of yourself, you often feel a sense of desperation. You are under constant pressure to feel validated, and almost anything can cause you to feel invalidated. A raised eyebrow, for example, may signal that the listener questions your entire worth as a person, not just the point you are trying to make. You crave affirmation and symbols of success or status.

A preoccupation with self stems from the constant pressure to experience validation and avoid invalidation. "Is this person attacking me?", "Don't they realize I'm an important person?" "I wonder if I'm coming across as stupid?" are questions asked by someone whose self worth seems frequently on the line. With such intense focus on the self, there is little room for others. A person, who repeatedly experiences shame and invalidation, is subject to many of the negative emotions associated with heart disease, such as depression, anxiety, and hostility.

Despite outward shows of bravado, a significant number of heart patients, have doubts about their ability to handle new situations, and are often frightened of new experiences. This is particularly true for me. I have to be brought, kicking and screaming to a new vacation destination. And just try to get me a new set of clothes for the trip. I'll fight you tooth and nail.

In addition to experiencing anxiety as a result of invalidation, a person who perceives that he has been treated poorly or unfairly, will often desire to strike back at those who invalidate him.

Sometimes this anger is turned inward. When anger is internalized, depression is often the result. As we will see, in a last ditch effort to right the scales, a person who feels "one down" may express his anger in self defeating ways: "I know what you want from me and I'll punish you by withholding it," or, "I'm mad at you so I won't take my medication."

JOURNAL REFLECTION – STEP 2

Describe a childhood experience that was extremely hurtful.

Do you crave approval, admiration, respect or attention? How often?

When you eavesdrop on your internal conversations, can you hear a Royal voice? Does it have an arrogant or humble tone?

STEP 3 – TAKE RESPONSIBILITY

> *Intense journey, huh? Don't worry, if you were able to look at shame and invalidation honestly, you're absolutely ready for the next step.*

When you take responsibility in your life,
you become free to change it.

Making mistakes is part of the natural plan for growing. You're expected to make mistakes and learn from them. In a natural growing progression, you try a strategy; it fails; you recognize that you didn't get what you intended; you adjust your strategy – until you succeed.

Think of a baby intent on standing:

ATTEMPT: baby tries to stand
FAILURE: baby plops right back down
ADJUSTMENT: baby makes another effort, slightly different this time (holding on to something)
FAILURE: (plop)
ADJUSTMENT: baby makes yet another strategy adjustment
FAILURE – ADJUSTMENT – FAILURE – ADJUSTMENT – FAILURE – ADJUSTMENT – FAILURE – ADJUSTMENT...
SUCCESS: baby stands

This trial and error process works perfectly for the baby. The baby accepts the outcome of its efforts without commentary. The baby does not look around for someone or something to blame for failure. The baby simply adjusts its behavior.

Unfortunately, as the baby grows up, something powerfully disruptive is interjected into an otherwise functional formula for growth. That powerful something is a judgment about who or what to blame for the "failure."

Failure is beneficial when it alerts you to change your approach. Your intention remains unchanged. The healthy developmental system breaks down when failure causes you to alter your intention. You change your intention once you add significance to your failure. This tiny mental addition is at the heart of what is wrong in the lives of many heart patients.

For example, you give up your intention to watch your weight because your previous diets failed. You tell yourself that you are a "weak willed" because you gained weight.

If you can admit that you had some part in your results, you free yourself from the false position of being a victim. Feelings of blame crowd out feelings of joy. Even when you are purposefully abused, you still get the final say in how you will hold that emotional trauma. Will you let the emotional burden hold you back or will you let yourself experience joy again?

Responsibility is about looking for your contribution to a situation, asking yourself: "How did I contribute to this situation? What part did I play? How did my behavior contribute to my current feelings?" When you can begin to see how you were instrumental in bringing about the situations in your life you are taking a monumental step toward health and well-being.

MY PERSONAL STEP 3

When I opened the Center for Cardiac Wellness, I noticed that many of my heart patients left treatment prematurely. When a heart patient withdraws from treatment after only a few sessions, he is sabotaging his own efforts to make necessary lifestyle changes. You can bet that the therapy process was perceived as too dangerous, and leaving the situation altogether seemed to be the least detrimental alternative for the patient.

What causes him to short circuit his good intentions is the threatened breakthrough of painful emotions. He would be unaware that therapy was threatening his defenses. His only awareness would be that the therapy was either too time consuming, too costly, or too impractical. Rather than see himself as being responsible for leaving treatment against advice, the "blame" was projected onto the therapist. The therapist might be regarded as too interested in money, too young, too old, too talkative or not talkative enough. Missing would be any recognition from the patient that he felt threatened or anxious about some of the areas being explored in therapy, or the therapy process itself. These thoughts and feelings remain unconscious.

Perhaps the heart patient begins to get a glimpse of what he missed growing up. A caring therapist who listens to the patient and doesn't criticize, has empathy for the patient's feelings, can be a threat to a person who has not experienced this kind of relationship anywhere in his life. Feelings of shame and deprivation may threaten to break through attempts to keep these painful feelings buried.

The other day one of my patients, who happens to be a nurse, described an incident with one of her heart patients. He apparently had a major heart event because he failed to take his medications. He stated that he didn't take his medications because he was mad at his cardiologist for not being as available to him as he had wished. This was an example of projecting responsibility for taking medication from himself to the cardiologist.

In the above situation, the patient may have been reminded of earlier experiences where as a child, he was dependent upon a caregiver who was frequently unavailable. The painful feelings associated with these experiences may have been rekindled when the doctor was unavailable. A heart patient may experience intense feelings which derail his good intentions, not unlike individuals diagnosed with Posttraumatic Stress Syndrome.

OBSTACLE 3: WE ARE OUR GENES

> *It is not easy to acknowledge that you were instrumental in bringing about certain situations in your life. Sometimes you flat out want to deny it. Watch out! You just encountered an obstacle.*

More and more research indicates that social and emotional factors play a significant part in the development of heart disease – that they are on par with traditional risk factors such as family history. It is not true that "This can't be helped." You *do* have control in the outcome of your health.

"This is not a good start for heart surgery", I told myself as I watched workmen with hardhats carrying sheetrock walk past me in the hallway. I was only 54 years old and had just said painful goodbyes to my wife before I was whisked away by a nurse and parked in a hallway outside the operating room. I was scared to death. My wife was only 40 and my son was just 6. What if quadruple by-pass surgery didn't work and I died on the operating table?

I could hear the banging and nail guns further down the hall, as the hospital was apparently being renovated. Left alone with my thoughts, in the middle of a construction site, I became increasingly anxious. I tried to reassure myself that I would survive the operation. After all, my father had identical procedure years before and did quite well. Still, I couldn't believe that I was being treated this way. Didn't they know I was a Doctor? With as much authority as I could muster in a hospital gown, I finally demanded that one of the construction workers find a nurse. When the nurse appeared, I demanded some Xanax to calm me down.

This accomplished, I was wheeled into the operating room where I was confronted by a second challenge. There were two doctors who greeted me at the door, and asked if I would consent to an experimental coronary by-pass procedure. I lost it. "How could you ask me to do this *NOW*?" I screamed. "If I say no, what are you going to do, kill me?" Taken aback by my anger and distrust, the doctors reassured me that I would be OK even if I refused to be a guinea pig. (I refused.) They did take good care of me. But it wasn't enough.

It's been 11 years since my open heart surgery, and I am still haunted by it. I often think of my father's quadruple by-pass surgery. He too said his goodbyes with tears in his eyes; because he had doubts that he would survive the risky operation. I was glad that my father's heart surgery went well. The years that were added to his life gave us the opportunity to mend many fences. I smiled to myself as I wondered how my father would have handled the circumstances that I had faced in the operating room.

Understand that my father took nothing lying down. He was a fighter from the get go. And he was always on guard lest others take advantage of him. I could actually picture him catapulting off the gurney and storming out of the operating room in protest, the back of his hospital gown flapping in the breeze. He would be muttering something about law suits as he trampled over a few startled workmen in hard hats who happened to be in his way.

My father and I had near identical surgical procedures at almost exactly the same age. My father and I were also similar in other important ways. We were distrustful, stubborn, competitive, and arrogant – characteristics highly influenced by social and emotional factors. We both became successful psychologists and authors. Genetics was only part of the picture for my father and me. I believe that our personalities and our experiences contributed to the formation of plaque in our arteries. Did we share a genetic predisposition towards coronary artery disease which was activated by psychosocial factors? I believe that to be the case.

Researchers have had success finding genes associated with heart disease. The problem is that individual genes rarely cause illness on their own. Instead, they tend to make people more susceptible. And in genetically mixed populations, the complex interaction among genes makes it hard to find the risky ones. Assuming that researchers will eventually find the genes associated with increased risk for heart disease, knowing that you have these genes will not, in and of itself, make much difference in your daily life. As we have seen, you have a *one in ten* chance of sustaining necessary lifestyle changes even when the diagnosis of coronary artery disease has been made and open heart surgery has occurred. There is no gene for following good advice. We cannot blame our genes, the phases of the moon, fate, or bad luck for how we turn out in life.

PROJECTION

Projection means placing the blame on others for things that are really your responsibility. You can observe this whenever you hear yourself say "_____ made me do it." Blaming others is so popular a defense that it has become almost an art form. "I wouldn't have to drink so much if I was married to an understanding person," might be one individual's refrain. Another might conclude that his boss, mother, neighbor, the weather, or the phases of the moon are at fault. "I could have been a contender," (if it weren't for _____.)" "Why should I be the one who has to change when I'm not the one who is at fault?"

RATIONALIZATION

Your inner voice will offer you wonderful ways to excuse your behaviors. "A few extra pounds won't kill you. You are entitled to a little pleasure." The inner voice is not above transforming reality to minimize your troublesome feelings. By rationalizing, you invent a socially acceptable and seemingly logical explanation for actions that can put you on the operating table.

AVOIDANCE

Did you ever see the commercials where a person does something embarrassing and the voiceover says, "Ever wish you could get away?" That situation is easy to identify with because we have all had miserably uncomfortable moments – moments when we would love to get away.

When you were a kid and did something wrong, you knew you were going to get punished. You wanted to get away not only to escape the punishment you felt was inevitable, but to escape the painful feelings of apprehension and dread as well. The dread might have been too much for you to bear. Your mind figured out a way for you to escape by imagining a more pleasant future or remembering a more palatable past.

As an adult our course of escape takes many forms. We can physically fly away to another place. We can dull the painful feelings by drowning them in alcohol, drugs, or comfort foods. We can distract ourselves by watching a good movie or keeping busy. And we can bury the pain altogether by refusing to think about it or feel anything.

I will never forget looking over at my son and seeing him clench his eyes shut as we were on the "Indiana Jones" ride in Disneyworld. In retrospect he was too young for that experience as my wife and I underestimated the ride's intensity. He tried valiantly to enjoy the ride, but as his fear mounted, he was forced to shut down his experiences.

Adults do this as well, but rather than literally shutting our eyes, we don't acknowledge our feelings. We repress what we can't stand. Our present moment is obliterated by a process that is outside our control.

When a painful memory is about to break through to awareness, an alarm goes off. Typically, you feel intense anxiety. Many heart patients attempt to stifle the alarm by destructive behaviors which are damaging to health. Overeating, drugs, and alcohol are some of the ways that people numb themselves.

The problem is that we can't get rid of unwelcome thoughts or feelings in the same way that we can get rid of things. If we don't like the movie, we can walk out of the theatre. But if we don't like our anxiety... Whatever we do to try to squash it, actually ends up intensifying it. As a coping strategy, trying to avoid your painful feelings by distraction, suppression, rationalization, or anesthesia just doesn't work. It's like trying not to think of a yellow Volkswagen.

JOURNAL REFLECTION – STEP 3

Who or what do you blame for your heart condition?
What are your favorite excuses to justify unhealthy behaviors?
How do you escape from painful feelings like worry or sadness?

STEP 4 – ACCEPTANCE BEGINS THE PROCESS OF HEALING

It is powerful just to recognize that you do sometimes avoid taking responsibility in your life. You've given yourself some breathing room. In order to begin healing those old wounds, read on.

Accepting your painful experiences begins to resolve the hurt.

You have come to the point in your journey where it's time to change the things you can change. You recognize harmful behaviors and toxic environments and you want no part of them. Getting out from under abuse and ending self-destructive habits will radically improve your life. So will acceptance of those things that you cannot change.

Acceptance of something is not the same as putting up with it. It is neither condoning nor approving. There are events in life that are upsetting to you that are beyond your control. Loved ones die. Your grief is normal and healthy. You feel the sadness, and you acknowledge that you are hurt. You accept your experience.

In a healthy life progression: You're born. You suffer hurt feelings growing up. (We all do). Your painful experiences become part of your history. You accept them. You resolve the hurts by facing them. You let people know how you feel. You learn from your painful experiences. They help you form healthy values. Your values guide your decisions. You adopt a healthy lifestyle. You live a long and fruitful life.

Suffice it to say that it didn't go that smoothly in your life progression *so far*. The point where you wandered off the path was at accepting what you felt in those painful experiences. "If it hurt back then, why would I want to dredge it up again?" The payoff comes at the next stage of the progression: resolution. Resolution of painful experiences means that the experiences are brought into your awareness and used to help you form your wisdom and character.

Remember your objective (being able to maintain a heart healthy lifestyle). Pain that remains unresolved has the power to ruin your life. You begin resolving pain by looking at it. Simply by examining an old emotional wound, you reduce its ability to hurt you.

Some feelings are not so easy to acknowledge. There are old wounds you just don't want to deal with. Try taking a baby step: Simply say, "Yes, that did happen to me." The next (bigger) baby step is answering the question, "How did that make you feel?" If you can flip through your painful memory album and make a caption for each item, you are striding through Step 4.

MY PERSONAL STEP 4

As a child, I could not show my anger without getting severely punished. Nor could I allow myself to experience sadness without putting an additional burden on my already stressed mother. Whenever feelings like anger or depression threatened to break through my attempts to suppress them, I would get anxious and fearful.

When a muscle doesn't get used, it atrophies. Likewise, if you don't feel your emotions, after a while, you loose touch with your emotions. Over time you loose the capacity to feel anger. It took nearly all the courage I could muster to admit to myself that I had a problem recognizing my feelings. From that point I could begin to resolve them.

Remember back before CDs? There were vinyl records you had to handle very carefully. If you got a scratch on one, the needle would skip to that scratch and etch the flawed track even deeper.

Etched in our memories, as on old records, are painful unresolved experiences. They were recorded because they were important. But, because they weren't resolved, we keep replaying those tracks – the same unresolved experiences – over and over.

One of my patients, Samantha, grew up with a father who withdrew in the face of conflict. Despite his own difficult past, her father was a successful businessman. Samantha thought he didn't care; she thought he didn't love her. Samantha went on a mission. "Let's see if I can get my father to pay attention to me." To her dismay, every outrageous action of hers met with non – reaction or intellectual interpretation from him. He just withdrew further, until one day he left altogether. Samantha blamed herself of course. Even though she knew he was unhappy with her mother, Samantha believed that if her father had really loved her he would have stayed.

Samantha was very angry at her father, but loved him too. She couldn't risk driving him further away by displaying her feelings – her sadness and her anger. She couldn't face her painful feelings. They became a record. Whenever something in the present reminded her of this unresolved pain, the broken record would play. As an innocent child, Samantha learned a coping mechanism from her father. When you are faced with conflict, swallow your feelings and withdraw. Suppress those hurtful feelings; don't experience them. You can always eat your way out of the pain.

If we resist facing our pain, our pain persists. If it is conflict that we fear most, conflict will always show up for us. If you are not willing to have it, you got it. The only way out of this mess is to accept what is. Accept that conflict frightens you. Be willing to experience the fear. While you're dancing to that broken record, you're not moving forward. You're not solving the problem. Writing about pain helps. Talking about it helps.

We can change only what can be changed. We can accept what can't be changed (the past). We don't have to accept abuse or alcoholism, but we can accept the painful feelings that accompany abuse. We can accept our desire to zone out when we are conflicted. But we don't have to act on our desire. We do have the capacity to change the record.

My wife is such a great role model; she taught me how to be angry! She demonstrated that you can be angry and then get over it. What a concept! You didn't have to implode and people didn't have to get annihilated (necessarily) when you got angry. You could get angry and live another day. You could still love someone who was just angry at you. And they could still love you after they were angry with you. She replaced my old record with a new one.

OBSTACLE 4: KEEP UP WITH THE JONESES

> *Acceptance really is the starting point of healing. You've come far to get to this point. You may be tempted to look around and see how you're doing compared to...Oops! – watch out for the obstacle; it's a mean one!*

Advertising and business interests bombard you with the myth that material possessions will bring you satisfaction. There aren't enough houses, boats, and cars to fill the void of what's really missing – if what's really missing is a lack of self worth. You get true self worth by handling issues, not by having things. Real satisfaction comes from self discipline and mastery.

THE "GREEN-EYED MONSTER"

Underneath the royal voice is envy – a sense of lack, a feeling of depletion. It is brought on by the perception that something is missing in oneself. It is the result of unfavorably comparing oneself to others' success, their reputation, their possessions, their luck, and their qualities. An envious person feels deprived a good deal of the time; he doesn't have enough money, can't get enough attention, isn't respected or acknowledged enough by his kids. Feeling deprived often sets up a sense of entitlement in people. It's as if the deprived person says "I have suffered too much. Now it's my turn to get special treatment."

Envy is the inevitable result of growing up in an invalidating environment – one which calls into question the entire worth of the person, not just his deeds. The envious person feels in a one-down position to start with, and has to prove to himself and to others that he is worthwhile. Ultimately, envy is about self hate. Self hate makes it downright impossible to sustain a healthy lifestyle.

Anger and envy can make you want to seek revenge on someone for making you feel empty or deprived. In order to be one-up on the envied one, revenge-minded heart patients may withhold their own joy or refuse to engage in health sustaining behaviors. These kinds of behaviors give the heart patient a kind of victory, but it is a hollow victory because it is at his own expense.

By way of retaliating for feeling one-down, you may try to give the sources of your envy as much grief as possible. Or you may say that the grapes are sour, rather than admit they are craved.

Envious people are likely to have a list of grievances. Grievances act like scar tissue covering up old emotional wounds. Every desire is looked at by comparison. Not only do you not have what you desire, someone else does have it – that rubs salt in your wounds. The human mind is automatically wired to compare things. Where we go wrong is in putting a judgment or evaluation on the comparison. I don't have what I want; she does; (judgment: that's wrong) I'm envious. We make significance out of what is just fact. We compound the problem by punishing – either the source or ourselves.

The green eyed monster feeds on self hate. Self hate can be remedied by learning to see yourself in a more favorable light. Get in touch with the unique person you are. Ask those people who love you, what it is that they truly value about you.

- Is it your sense of humor? – quick wit?
- Your creativity?
- Irreverence?
- The fact that you can be counted on when the going gets rough?
- The little boy underneath the kingly façade?
- The part of you that is trying to be better?

Enhancing your self esteem is the antidote for self hate and envy. You're unlikely to be envious that others have food on the table when you have just eaten a delicious meal.

You can feel better about yourself by increasing your achievements or reducing your expectations. In my experience, it is harder for heart patients to reduce their expectations. We are very talented and successful people who, despite our achievements, fall short of our own demands and requirements.

I remember feeling bad about not having the things that many of the other children had. At the time I wasn't able to label my feelings as envy. All I knew was that, in comparison to me, the other kids had fathers who were available to play football, mothers who were home and cooked great meals; bikes that didn't break down all the time; and money to play the pinball machines at the local hangout. Some of my friends were better athletes, more popular with the girls, or smarter. None of this was lost upon me.

As an adult, I was envious of others' status and success, as well as their possessions. If a colleague graduated from an Ivy League School, or had achieved some professional award, I inevitably compared myself to him and came up short. If a friend was able to purchase a beautiful house, rather than feel good for him, the feeling I had to stuff down was envy.

No matter how many awards I received, or how many things I owned, it was never enough for me. Heart patients like me feel a sense of emotional deprivation that can only be filled through intangibles, such as love, appreciation, and inner satisfaction from work. These qualities aren't obtained through sheer force of will, or by accumulating material possessions; if they come, it is through self esteem.

JOURNAL REFLECTION – STEP 4

Who do you compare yourself with unfavorably? Why?

What do others truly love about you? Why?

What new activities would enhance your self esteem?

STEP 5 – CLEANSE YOUR MIND

> *What a relief to recognize that you can get satisfaction from within. This "clearing" in your way of thinking is the perfect place from which to take the next step.*

Cleanse your mind by letting go of your harmful emotions.

Your mind is now open to new possibilities. You're starting to discern your helpful inner guidance. You've begun taking responsibility for your behavior. And you are accepting the feelings you've experienced in order to resolve your pain. It is time to take the next step toward your well-being and heart health – letting go of your harmful emotions.

Being able to recognize and experience a wide range of emotions is healthy. Knowing that you're disappointed, angry, or embarrassed in a situation gives you direction for handling it effectively. Problems arise when you don't recognize and deal with the uncomfortable emotions you feel. If you don't learn to work with your emotions they will work against you. Harmful emotions can wreak havoc on your body and spoil your relationships.

All children have to deal with hurtful experiences. If they are lucky, there are people in their lives who can soothe their pain and teach them how to cope. With guidance, children learn to identify their feelings and to process them in an emotionally healthy way. Some are not so lucky. They don't learn and grow from their pain; it gets mishandled. When children aren't taught good coping skills they often deal with pain in an emotionally unhealthy way.

In an unsupportive environment, children are likely to try anything to keep their pain at bay. They repress or bury their thoughts, memories, and feelings – anything associated with painful experiences. This strategy inevitably backfires.

Repression of pain begins a vicious cycle: When you first went through the painful experience, you felt you couldn't bear to face your thoughts and feelings about it. You decided that those memories were too hot to handle so you didn't handle them – you buried them (alive). Then you began to worry, "What if they were to rise up from the grave!?" You worry turns to fear. Now you've got an additional problem. You're standing over the grave of the dormant pain (from the thought, memory, or feeling), terrified of experiencing that pain. It has taken on a demonic aspect – you now dread feeling it.

It gets worse. It takes constant vigilance and effort to keep painful memories from reaching consciousness. This effort is exhausting. You're already edgy from fear. Something happens that vaguely reminds you of the buried memory. Your worst fear is happening: The demon is rising from the grave to make you feel the pain. You panic. You explode, attack, weep, whatever. You are not reacting to the situation at hand, you are protecting yourself *at any cost* from reliving that pain.

The trigger for these outbursts can be anything – whatever conjures up memories that you are avoiding dealing with. A look can remind you of a put-down that hurt. A certain laugh can be associated with extreme embarrassment.

You fly off the handle over the littlest thing. When someone cuts in front of you when you're driving, you lay on the horn, curse them, and jack up your blood pressure. You know your reaction is disproportionate, but you can't seem to control it. Or someone tells you "No way" when you make a request. Now is the time to ask yourself what painful experience in your past does "No way" remind you of. It's your response to these old repressed feelings that causes you to overreact, not the current situation.

This calls for some tough soul-searching, but you'll find the hard work worthwhile. Until you recognize your previous injury, you will be triggered to protect against feeling it at any cost. The best defense (the only healthy defense) is a good offense. Start digging up those demons and discover that their ability to hurt you fades in the light of your bold examination.

MY PERSONAL STEP 5

One day one of my patients, Rodger, was devastated when he hit a weak shot playing golf. When one of his golf associates jokingly called him "Susan", he almost walked off the golf course in "disgrace". Nobody had a clue as to how his stepfather had abused him, and therefore how exquisitely sensitive he was about his manhood.

Even Rodger was puzzled by his extreme reaction to being teased. He was unable to connect his childhood experiences with his behavior on the golf course. Rodger had buried painful memories of being humiliated by his step father. Shame and rage were the attendant feelings associated with the memory. These feelings were also buried. Once he was able to talk about these experiences and express his feelings, he became less reactive and less likely to be triggered. Rodger had tamed one of his demons.

Whenever my wife called to tell me that she would be late coming home, I would raid the refrigerator even though I knew this was damaging to me. Why did I do this? For me, her coming home late triggered countless times when I was alone as a child because my mother had to be away working to support the family. I was angry at my mother and angry at my wife for "deserting" me. But since I could not express my anger at either person whom I depended upon for love, I turned the anger inward. I learned to prevent that particular trigger from setting me on a path of self-destructive behavior. This is how I got past it.

First: I had insight. (I realized that I was revisiting my past hurt in my present situation.)

Second: I realized that the two events were distinct. (My wife's lateness was not the same as my mother's absence.)

Third: I recognized that my old memory elicited painful feelings. (I felt anxiety and sadness when my mother was away working.)

Fourth: I reasoned that punishing my wife (or myself) wasn't appropriate. (My wife's lateness was not the source of my sadness.)

Fifth: I choose healthy ways to deal with these feelings. (I shared my experience with my wife.)

Sixth: I took action to sustain my healthy choice. (I asked my wife for support in not repeating the old pattern. Now she reminds me not to be sad when she's going to be late.)

OBSTACLE 5: BITE YOUR TONGUE

> *How long has it been since you've had true peace of mind? It certainly is a commodity worth cherishing, perhaps guarding. Uh oh. Yep, you spotted it ahead – an obstacle.*

Normal feelings come and go. When we don't allow their expression, we can make them toxic. Toxic feelings fester underneath the rubble in the wake of painful experiences. Toxic waste can prevent us from getting the love we need and living the life of our dreams. We need to express our painful feelings not bite our tongues. We need to accept our experiences, even the painful ones to get what we really want.

Exposure to invalidating experiences creates additional problems for you. When you are threatened to your very core with extinction, you tend to fight as if your life depends upon it (maybe it does). When you hear messages as a child, that cut you deeply, like "You are lazy," or "Stupid," there is a part of you that wants to fight back in protest. It's the part of you that sticks your jaw out and says "No I'm not!" or "I'll show you!" or "You can't hurt me." Another part of you wants to guard against the possibility that these kinds of messages can ever hurt you again. This pattern continues into adulthood.

For me, "I'll show you," meant becoming a tennis champion in my local club, and captain of the Crew team in College. It meant overcoming multiple rejections every step of the way as I pursued a Doctorate in Psychology, and in securing post-doctoral training in various institutions. It meant chairing several professional groups. Finally, "I'll show you," meant becoming a successful Psychologist/Entrepreneur. My jaw is sticking out as I write this.

I have observed in many of my heart patients this same desire to prove themselves. There is a deep sense of pride and a steely resolve which seems to say to the world, "Go ahead, take your best shot." One of my heart patients witnessed the murderous behavior of her father. She decided then and there never to marry. She is over 70 years old, still single, and has stuck to her guns.

While true grit may have enabled my heart patients to achieve success in business, it is this same stubbornness that prevents them from achieving success in intimate relationships.

Life can be a scary prospect, but if you don't let down your guard you never develop. It would be like keeping your child under guard in the house because you're afraid he might get hurt. What are we guarding against? We are guarding against the experience of painful feelings. But some of those painful feelings have valuable messages attached. You need to remember the fear you felt lying on the operating table. If you keep guarding against feeling that pain, you won't learn from your experience.

It can be extremely difficult to let down your guard, particularly if you fear that your weakness could be exploited by your enemies. In making a bold choice to let down your guard despite your concerns, you are electing to be somebody other than who you have been – you choose to be trusting. This is hard to do because you are used to who you have been your whole life. After all, you have accomplished a lot. Is there anyone who could easily say, "I have been wrong my whole life?" Better the devil you know...

TOXIC EMOTIONS

Anxiety

Given the stresses of modern life, it is normal to experience occasional anxiety. However, if you are dealing with heart disease, you suffer from persistent worry and tension that is worse than most people feel from time to time. The high level of anxiety can make even ordinary activities difficult. When I'm preoccupied with paying the bills, it is very difficult for me to take the dog for a walk.

Although many people may realize that their anxiety is excessive or unwarranted, they are unable to simply "snap out of it." Of course, you can guard against the experience of anxiety (or any other experience) by hiding under your bed, but then you will not have lived much of a life. The best way to deal with anxiety is to look at it as a signal that growth is ahead.

How Do You Know When You Are In An Anxious State?

Do you often feel edgy, restless, or keyed up? Do you tire easily? Do you have trouble concentrating? Are you irritable? Do you experience increased muscle tension? Do you have trouble sleeping? These are all signs of anxiety. One of my heart patients recently disclosed to me that he experienced each and every one of these states on a daily basis, yet he didn't recognize that he was anxious!

As a child, I experienced what I now know to be anxiety every day. Growing up in an environment that was chaotic and unpredictable was anxiety provoking. I remember being sick a lot as a kid, with symptoms that I realize were anxiety based. If, "Whenever you are afraid, just whistle a happy tune," had been my theme song, I would have been whistling most of the time. As an adult, I am still anxious a good deal of the time, despite my attempts at bravado.

Most of us like a certain degree or predictability, order and control. We devote our lives to sameness, habit, and familiarity as a source of stability and comfort. I have had several periods in my life where I ate the same lunch every day for years. I love my old clothes, my morning routines, and sticking with old friends. By rigidly adhering to habits, we can contain our anxiety somewhat.

Some heart patients know more about heart disease than their cardiologist does. They collect information to defend against feeling their anxiety. Their information gets used like a barrier to changing, rather than being used to change their behavior. Their intellect would be better applied in accepting and resolving the source of their anxiety rather than guarding against it.

For starters, how about at least accepting in principle that anxiety can be a good thing? Anxiety can cause you to move forward and evolve into someone new and enlivened. It is far more invigorating to welcome change and uncertainty with an adventurous spirit than it is to cower and stagnate behind your T.V. for hours on end. What you fear the most rarely happens anyway, so why get yourself in a tizzy?

Diminishing the Feeling of Anxiety

Say to yourself, "I'm willing to accept this." Decide to be with the experience of uncertainty. View anxiety as a sign that growth is ahead. Observe your thoughts, feelings, and actions as if you are a friendly but not overly concerned bystander:

"I am getting anxious now. How interesting! I wonder why this person/situation is making me anxious? On a scale of 1 to 10, how would I score my anxiety at this moment? Am I breathing slowly and normally?" By doing this you can watch the peaks and valleys of your anxiety and not be so effected by it.

Depression

That same invalidating environment which created envy and shame as by-products, sets up the conditions for depression as well. We re-experience depression whenever we are faced with reminders of what we felt was missing or lacking back then. There may be very little in the way of positive experience stored in our memory banks. Heart patients are characterized by having a diminished reserve energy capacity. There is little to draw from that can support and sustain us during lean times. We are already driving on empty. And it doesn't take much for us to run out of gas, and feel depleted.

Who me?

One problem that many of us have is that we don't always know when we are depressed. Do you often feel tearful, lethargic, worthless, indecisive? These are all signs of depression.

When I'm depressed I can't do much of anything. Still, there are things that help. Having a friend take you out; going to a movie; talking about what bothers you; communing with nature; helping someone else, for starters.

Anger

I find that I am most angry when I am in my kingly mode. As a king, the world should do as His Majesty commands. When the world doesn't operate in accordance with the wishes of His Majesty, the natural response is to get angry. So, arrogance is a certain trigger for anger, and we know that many patients struggling with heart disease are arrogant. Our shaky self esteem is supported when we carry a scepter and wear a crown.

Anger is most often related to your level of self esteem. When your self esteem is threatened, anger can be the result. No one likes to be attacked, diminished or criticized. Since many individuals with heart disease have experienced invalidation repeatedly as children, we are sitting ducks when it comes to being triggered by criticism.

Unmet expectations present another cause for anger. Whenever you believe that things should be a certain way and they turn out to be different, anger may be the result. For example, if you thought that your boss would give you a raise, only to find out that your pay is the same, you would get angry at your boss for not fulfilling your expectations.

The other day one of my patients came into my office still fuming about someone in the waiting room who was "eating like a pig" while somehow talking loudly on his cell phone. My patient was enraged by this inappropriate behavior. However, his high degree of upset was really related to his having "pigged out" himself earlier.

Whenever you perceive you have lost control of a situation (where you expected or demanded to have control), anger may erupt. Situations which invoke unwelcome feelings such as fear or frustration are often seen as occurring outside of your control. For example, you are driving along when suddenly a car passes you dangerously on the right. You have no control over what happened and no control over your racing heartbeat. You become angry and resentful because you assert that someone did something he shouldn't do. His actions serve to underscore your lack of control. A tightly-wound individual who craves control does not like his authority questioned, or his sense of security threatened.

How Can You Tell?

You can tell that you're angry by tuning in to your body. Are you grinding your teeth? Is your heart beating rapidly? Are your palms sweating? Certain situations may trigger you:

? Do you sense your heart pounding or your breath quickening when you find yourself in a slow line in traffic or at the bank or supermarket?

? If an elevator stops too long on the floor above you, are you likely to pound on the door, stomp your feet or clench your fist?

? When in the supermarket express line do you often count the items in the baskets of people ahead of you to be sure that they are not over the limit?

Although anger is naturally occurring and often a healthy response to threat or frustration, when it occurs too frequently or lasts too long anger becomes dangerous to health. The experience of anger can be reduced in frequency and intensity by changing how you think. Get rid of the "shoulds" in your self talk, and replace them with "coulds." "He should have given me a bonus," is a thought that can easily trigger anger in the event of a disappointment. Changing the statement to "He could have given me a bonus," opens up the possibility of different interpretations in the event of disappointment. Using "could" implies that there is more to the story; it allows you to reason with yourself and reduce your level of anger.

Upsets do not necessarily have to lead to anger. You could increase your tolerance for frustration by re-framing the situation. For example, consider that your teenager's messiness is good training for becoming less compulsive or rigid.

Accept that there are situations which are out of your control. It takes wisdom to "go with the flow," and accept what you cannot change. View yourself as an evolving person rather than a fixed entity. This will put you in a position to see all of your experiences as learning experiences, especially the difficult ones. You are here to fulfill your potential as a human being, and this means that there is always more to learn. Experience is the greatest teacher if you are open to it.

I have often asked myself, "What am I supposed to learn from my battles with heart disease? How can I put my experiences to good use?" I now see that I was in the perfect position to wrestle with these questions. As a Psychologist, I could understand the emotional factors that de-rail our best intentions to change – and I could write about them. As an arrogant king, I could learn firsthand the dangers of my stance, the origins of it, and the need to develop another side of my personality – and I could develop humility. As a rebellious individual, who fought hard against convention, I could learn what I had to do in order to step out of that role – and I could learn the benefits of surrendering to the heart felt advice of my doctors and family.

JOURNAL REFLECTION – STEP 5

How do you prove to others that you are a "somebody"?
What do you fear would happen if you let down your guard?
Which of the toxic emotions do you frequently experience?

STEP 6 – ACT WITH INTEGRITY

> *If you resolve the painful memories and feelings that plague you,*
> *you are free to act according to your own will. But how can you*
> *be sure that you'll act in ways that will bring you personal*
> *satisfaction and keep you healthy? You need a code to live by.*
> *You need to take the next step.*

When you act with integrity you can change your world.

The courageous journey you have taken to get to this point has stopped the steady progress of destructive behavior. Keep your eye on the target. You are intent on being that *one in ten* who is able to sustain a healthy lifestyle. It is time to begin taking steps toward constructive behaviors – choices that support your well-being.

Because you have shed bright light on them, you are aware of some of the things that trigger you to engage in unhealthy patterns of behavior. Exposure has broken their absolute control of you. You are no longer being run by these triggers; you can choose your response to them. This brings you to a critical juncture. How will you go about choosing wisely?

In order to make any choice, you must make decisions. By definition, decision means "cutting away" the alternatives. You cannot be decisive in your choice of direction until you are clear where you want to go. Clarity comes from examining your goals – the ones you make obvious and the ones you are careful to conceal. Honesty, at this step, will help get you what you really want.

Revealing the truth can be hard. You may be afraid that your honesty will lead to negative outcomes. If you admit that your lifestyle is not working for you, despite your desire to change, you may be exposing yourself to criticism. If you admit that your want to be healthy and yet do not take care of yourself, you may be subjected to guilt and condemnation. When you admit that you have disappointed loved ones with your behavior you risk feeling remorse for their grief.

In order to make wise decisions consistently, you need to have a well-defined code that works for you. Anyone can draw up a code of high standards, ethics, and principles of behavior – the hard part is following it. People don't follow lofty codes – not over the long run, anyway. If you are to generate a useful code (one that helps you make decisions) you will have to be honest with yourself.

Your code is built on the principles you choose to live by. Establishing principles to live by and living by these principles is living in integrity. Truth, honor, and reliability are elements of integrity. The origin of the term is "whole". It describes you as you were meant to be – a whole being. This includes your thoughts and actions, your memories, and the pain you've endured.

Your code is not a list of "Thou shalt…"'s. Only a code that is gentle and compassionate, encouraging and acknowledging to you will serve. Only a code formed by you, for you, will be sustainable. In order to live by your code and live in integrity, you have to tell the truth. You, and only you, can say what counts for you. *The truth shall set you free.* That's a decent payoff for your hard work.

MY PERSONAL STEP 6

At this point in my journey I could finally admit to myself that my lifestyle was killing me and that I had to change. I learned to see myself in a new light.

I realized that I had been stubborn. I told myself over and over again that this was a new day and that today I was going to embark upon a heart healthy lifestyle. One day turned into the next, and 10 years later I was still saying the same thing – waiting for the next day to begin changing.

I was too proud to ask for help. I prided myself on being independent and tough minded. I thought that asking for help was a sign of weakness, an admission of failure. Besides, I didn't know who to ask for help.

I was unaware of what was really going on inside my head. I couldn't hear the inner voice that kept urging me to do what I wanted without concern for the consequences to my health. I was unaware that painful childhood experiences were still running me. It's hard to tell the truth about something that you can't see. In order to avoid feeling toxic emotions such as anxiety, depression and envy, I developed an arrogant personality.

I was quick to make excuses for myself whenever I got off track. I had a hard day at the office. No one understands me. I kept getting triggered by the painful feelings I attempted to keep buried.

I couldn't see that I was afraid of intimacy. I couldn't trust anyone with my feelings and therefore could not allow myself to be vulnerable. I put up barriers between myself and others in self defense. I was unaware of how I had hurt others by my actions. Moreover, I did not really know how to be charitable with others; I was wholly caught up in my own gratification.

I was able to improve the odds that I could sustain a healthy lifestyle by being honest with myself. I started paying attention to my arrogant thoughts and behaviors. This paved the way for feelings of humility and appreciation to show up.

I have become a role model for my patients. I tell the truth to them and to myself. In short, I became an authentic person.

BECOMING AUTHENTIC

Becoming authentic entails the profound task of avoiding self deception and hidden agendas. Authenticity requires courage, being vulnerable, sticking your neck out. To help determine if you are being authentic, ask yourself the following question:

Do people know you for who you are?

When all your cards are on the table, it's a lot easier for others to play with you. Self disclosure prolongs life by creating intimacy.

BARRIERS TO AUTHENTICITY

Fear of rejection is a major barrier to authenticity. Many heart patients were trained or conditioned by parents and teachers to "fit in" or be a "good child." Their personalities were more or less imposed upon them. Someone with a conditioned personality does not adapt well in a rapidly changing world. Not knowing who he is, he cannot look within for answers. The best he can do is to ask others, "What should I do?" Then he must follow with, "Is what I'm doing acceptable?" It is a vicious cycle – he's now vulnerable to rejection.

Contrast this with what an authentic person does. He has learned from his experiences and has formed his own conclusions. He is a self-discovered person.

A good to way to get rid of your fear of rejection is to face your fear – go out and self disclose. You can't wait for the fear to go away before you act. You must do it in order for the fear to go away. Pushing through the fear of self disclosure is less damaging to the heart than pretending that you are what you are not. To be authentic we must recognize and handle our fear of being known. Intimacy and healing depend upon our success in laying down our facades.

OBSTACLE 6: LOGIC SAVES THE DAY

Acting with integrity is its own reward. It's starting to look as if things will go your way after all. You're back in control. Great, for now. But what about that tiny spark that's hovering above your powder keg of emotions!? You know – the times you go from elated to ballistic in a heartbeat. You've arrived at an obstacle.

It is well understood that your thinking determines what you feel, and what you feel determines what you do. If you think someone's out to get you, you feel threatened and you may fight or flee – a perfectly reasonable course of action. In law, medicine, and education, logic and reason are essential. Other times, just the reverse is true. What you feel dictates what you do. Your thoughts follow to make sense of your behaviors. If the tiger is about to attack, you feel threatened and dive for cover without thinking. Thinking would slow you down. Once you're safe and sound you will have the luxury of trying to make sense of what happened. Sometimes your reasoning can kill you.

THE "RATIONAL" MIND

We are most conscious of the rational mind when we ponder, reflect, or think through issues. We heart patients (and our doctors) are masters of this domain. We like to share our thoughts and opinions but prefer to keep our feelings more private. We keep generating thoughts, as many as 60,000 a day it has been estimated.

Thoughts we are attached to gel into beliefs. A belief is a group of thoughts that we accept as absolutely true. Beliefs are not dependent upon facts or scientific evidence to exist. Yet they can influence our perceptions and interpretations and can limit our ability to maneuver in the world. We have already visited several beliefs (obstacles) that took us on a wild goose chase and kept us away from the path to heart health.

What if you said to yourself "My anxiety is too much to bear?" If you become so attached to this thought that it becomes a reality, you will ultimately constrict your life so as not to experience this feeling. You have elevated a thought to a belief – and then acted on that belief. This (untrue) belief influences the way you live your life. Instead, what if the thought was "My anxiety is a sign that growth is ahead?" Your behavior would turn out to be quite different.

It's hard to get the distance we need to see that our thoughts only *represent* reality. Lacking accurate perspective, we make the mistake of defining ourselves and our experiences in accordance with our limiting thoughts. In fact, our health depends on the nature of our limiting thoughts and the ability to balance our thoughts with our emotions.

EMOTIONAL INTELLIGENCE

It didn't seem to matter how much education I had, or how smart I was, when I was in the grip of emotion. What mattered was my ability to handle my emotions, my emotional intelligence. Unfortunately, I learned I had very little emotional intelligence and the heart patients I had been counseling were in the same sinking boat.

To understand what I mean, it is necessary to know the difference between Emotional Intelligence and Intelligence as we usually think about it (a number signifying your I.Q., or Intelligence Quotient). Intelligence Quotient (I.Q.) is a measure of intellectual capacity to handle information and complex situations. The ability to pay attention, concentrate, solve puzzle-like problems, and comprehend are some of the areas that comprise I.Q. In general, my heart patients would score high on an I.Q. test. Their rational minds were exquisite.

Emotional Intelligence (E.Q.) is the ability to recognize and regulate emotions, both in you and in others. A person with a high emotional intelligence is aware of his feelings, thoughts and values; he can calm himself and others. Such a person is not prone to flying off the handle, rationalization, or exhibiting situational values. These people have rich emotional lives. They are comfortable with themselves and others. Individuals like this are not only well adjusted, they live longer. For example, people who manage moods well, a characteristic of emotional intelligence, are 50 times more likely to be alive 15 years later, than those with low self-regulation skills.

Because people with emotional intelligence are self-aware, they have fewer blind spots than most people, and can draw upon a broad range of emotions and personality traits to solve problems. Individuals fitting this personality profile are actually made stronger by extremely difficult circumstances.

The idea that you can be measured along the E.Q. dimension is a relatively new one, at least in comparison with scoring I.Q. The E.Q. measure was quantified as it became increasingly obvious that there were some very smart people, as measured by the I.Q. test, who were failures when it came to dealing with emotions.

They couldn't discern when they were angry, depressed, or ashamed. They were unaware when they were being defensive; they often misread what others were feeling. They were unable to calm themselves down or persist at a task when the going got rough.

It seemed to come as a shock to my patients, that I knew their feelings better than they did. I might say, "John, are you aware that you are angry right now? Your face is red, the veins are bulging out of your head and neck, your jaw is clenched, you're sitting at the edge of your seat and your fists look ready to deck someone." Amazingly, John could be unaware that he was angry despite the evidence. Once John learned to recognize his anger, he could discover the source of it. He learned that he became angry at the thought of being unfairly treated.

Preferring facts (data, information), patients like John seemed rattled when we began to explore their feelings. Many saw feelings as irrelevant or annoying and wanted to get on with what they perceived was more reasonable – more facts, information, and directions as to exactly what I thought they should do.

As I spent more time with my patients I began to see the myriad ways that they attempted to suppress, reduce, diminish, control, or counteract their painful feelings. Whether they numbed themselves in front of a T.V., exercised obsessively, worked long hours, ate or drank too much, or rationalized or denied what was going on, it was clear that they just didn't want to feel their pain. Not that anyone wants to feel pain…but if you continually suppress the source of your pain, you cannot learn how to diminish it. How did we get this way?

HIDE YOUR FEELINGS

As children, you were taught that you should be able to control your feelings. "Big boys don't cry," was a message that I heard frequently. Besides, grownups seemed to handle their feelings pretty well. I never thought for a minute that my father could be scared, or my mother depressed. As a child, I wasn't yet able to see the subtle signs that my parents really had feelings like me. I thought that I had to control or hide my feelings like all the adults around me. Somehow I thought that people who expressed their feelings were weak and couldn't do any better.

Most of my heart patients are successful in the real world. They have often achieved good positions at work, have raised families, and live in relative comfort. They accomplished all this by being somewhat controlling of events and people. It is little wonder that individuals with success controlling the world outside the body, would attempt to control feelings as well. For the "successful" heart patient, feelings are often a nuisance and a distraction to be controlled by the rational mind.

Like many professional people, I took great pride in my intellectual skills. After all, I struggled for many years in college to gain the knowledge that I now have. So it came as quite a shock to me when I discovered that I had overvalued my rational mind and ignored the impact of emotions on my behavior. In terms of balance, when we overvalue our intellect, we undervalue our emotions.

The imbalance also means that we underestimate our emotions. I had no idea how powerful my emotions could be and how I was at their mercy. Following doctor's orders, eating the right foods, exercising, and keeping myself relatively calm in the face of severe stress, turned out to be more a function of how well I handled emotions, and less about being reasonable. I found out that my emotional mind often swamped my rational mind. When the tiger attacks, reason is worthless – better just fight or flee.

EMOTIONAL HIJACKING

Our emotions, with their powerful impulses, and sometimes illogical actions, seem to come on suddenly – more quickly than reasoning can unfold. We heart patients are often puzzled by our emotional reactions, and at times may not even be aware that emotions drove us to behave in certain ways. Who among us has not been hijacked by a state of craving or aversion that we did not understand?

Heart patients are sitting ducks when it comes to unexpected, unwelcome emotions. We often don't recognize them, can't name them, and have little skill in handling them. Our minds are frequently out of balance. Like combat veterans diving for cover whenever they hear a loud noise, heart patients are often geared up for battle when no real threat exists.

One of my patients, Terry, reported that his temper would flare any time that he perceived that he was being told what to do. He hated the feeling of being talked down to as if he were a little boy. If his wife asked him to pick up something from the store, Terry would interpret her request as a direct order, and then flip out. Any request by his children, was met immediately with a "no." Terry placed the origin of his sensitivity and over- reactions, to having been dominated and controlled by his father. No matter how many times he tried not to react like his father, Terry found himself helpless to behave in any other way. Terry was a frequent victim of emotional hijacking.

In order to interrupt the chain of events that leads to an emotional hijacking, you must be present to your experience in the moment. This means that you can't suppress your thoughts or feelings but instead must allow them, whatever they are. You must become more familiar with your inner world--the pattern of your thoughts, feelings and impulses. Just knowing this interrupts the chain of reactive thoughts and feelings. Once the chain is broken, you are free to choose consciously how you will behave; whether to give in to unhealthy behaviors, or sustain a healthy lifestyle.

The problem for us heart patients is that we are not present to our experiences very often. We rarely know our own feelings, have repressed many of our painful memories, and have developed habits of numbing ourselves to present experiences that are connected to these painful memories. "Those who forget history are doomed to repeat it." Likewise, without an understanding of how our painful experiences affect us, we are reduced to trying again and again to correct our mistakes.

BECOMING EMOTIONALLY INTELLIGENT

There are things you can do which help:

- Try to put your emotions in words. People who are at risk for heart disease are often unable to identify when they are angry or sad, or even anxious.
- Get in touch with your "shoulds" and replace them with wants, wishes and desires, in order to give yourself more choice in your life.
- When under stress, stop what you are doing and try to remember a time when you felt love, care, or appreciation. The feeling of joy or delight is incompatible with the feeling of stress.
- Don't presume that people can read your mind. Share your thoughts (appropriately).
- Counterbalance a tendency towards seriousness with a spirit of playfulness.

These tips are useful *only* to the degree that they are practiced regularly. You are as likely to create transformational changes by simply reading a list of tips, as you are to improve your golf game by reading a book.

JOURNAL REFLECTION – STEP 6

Do people know you for who you are? Explain.

Are you more of are a "feeling" person (relying on your emotions) or more of a "thinking" person (relying on facts and data)?

What are the principles you chose to live by – your personal code?

STEP 7 – LIVE IN THE MOMENT

> *Knowing that you can slow or stop the progression of an emotional meltdown is such a relief! It can restore your confidence and make you want to get out there and participate in life again. You want to do everything you've put off from yesterday and plan tomorrow. But what about now, right now? Now is the time for the next step.*

It is in the moment that you access true vitality.

Of course you are living in this moment…and this one… The question is, "Where is your attention?" The human mind is an amazing thing; it allows you to tune in or to zone out. According to Eckhart Tolle, author of *The Power of Now*, the mind focuses mostly on the past and the future. Rarely are we here, paying attention now. Being present takes intention.

Having a past, a present, and a future awareness is normal and useful. The mind's focus on the past gives you a sense of continuity and identity. Its focus on the future ensures your continued survival and enables you to seek fulfillment some day. Of these three time contexts, the present is the least often visited. Your mind flits through the present on its way to past, then to the future, then back to the past… Unchecked, your mind is as reactive as a pin ball bouncing off the bumpers. "What if…? – Remember when…? – Oh, no! This must mean…!"

The vast majority of thoughts, feelings, and urges that waft through our minds in every moment are often outside our awareness. The conscious effort to focus awareness is known as "mindfulness." In a state of mindfulness it can feel as if time has slowed down. Details become apparent. Your attention is fully engaged in what you focus on. A peaceful quality often accompanies this state of awareness. It has been described as "out of mind."

In order to get the most out of life, you need to be present to the greatest extent possible. This implies being aware of what is going on in and around you in each moment. In "perfect awareness" you are wholly present in the moment and hear no distracting internal chatter. Athletes describe this as "being in the flow."

As you aspire to experience more and more moments of perfect awareness, you can notice the degree to which you are present to what's going on in any given moment. This does not mean that every present moment is wonderful. It is just as it is. The problem comes when we judge the moment and find fault with it. We are not willing for it to be the way it is; we want to experience something else. We're OK with the "good" moments but we don't want the "bad" moments to exist.

Judgment is one of the enemies of a peaceful mind. We make ourselves more miserable when we try to resist what is. What we resist persists in our worlds and provides us with an unending source of irritation and grief.

The counterpart to judgment is acceptance. Not approval or agreement, just acknowledgment that it is the way it is. You witness the experience, the feeling, the situation; you do not react to it or judge it. Having this attitude contributes countless benefits to our lives. It directly influences peace of mind – the mind which serves the healthy body.

My Personal Step 7

I have found an especially useful way to bring myself into the moment when I discover that I'm caught up in a drama of mental ping-pong. It is focusing on my breathing. When I make a conscious effort to breathe slowly and normally, the results are amazing. I can go from fantasy, with attendant anxiety, to reality, with attendant peace, in the space of a breath!

Recognizing when I'm not present is another great way to bring myself back to the moment.

————————

Ask yourself:

_____   Do I spend a lot of my time thinking about how things were?
_____   Do a lot of my sentences begin with, "What if…?"
_____   Do I have the feeling my life is on hold?
_____   Do I make extensive To Do lists?
_____   Do I often feel a sense of aliveness and joy?

The statements that describe you indicate your orientation – past, present, or future. Why is this important? Because to the extent that you are living in the past or the future, you are not living in the present. And it is only in the present that you can choose a healthy lifestyle.

What happens when your mind is in the past? Well, you are busy looking over your shoulder for the next threat to come your way. Exhaustion, depletion, distress, and negative feelings like depression or guilt are some of your companions. Unhealthy behaviors you employ to quash these feelings may increase your risk of heart disease.

What happens when your mind is in the future? Regardless of how much you do or how much you earn, it is never enough. You keep hoping for happiness that never comes. Relaxing with nothing to do is not possible for you, since you are being "non-productive." You are under constant worry about what might happen and knock yourself out trying to cover all the possible contingencies you imagine.

The only place that you can be conscious and aware is in the present moment. In the now is where you feel a certain level of peace and satisfaction. This is where healing can take place. It is the only place from which real choice can occur.

When you're in the moment, you're in the flow. You are absorbed in what you are doing. You are not thinking about it, judging it, or evaluating it. You are simply living it. You lose track of time. Is there anything wrong in the present? The answer is, "No. There is nothing wrong in this instant." It is only when you add judgment to the moment that things become not OK. When you're in your mind you are not in the present. You can be feeling bad because of something that happened in the past. You can remember some painful event for example. Or you can be feeling bad because you are imagining some event that hasn't yet taken place – some future event that you are worried about. But then is not now.

One way to access the present is to get in touch with what you love. Doing what you love puts you in the flow. It increases your energy and your vitality. The enthusiasm you experience from doing what you love can fuel your ability to make wise choices.

19

OBSTACLE 7: WHAT'S DONE IS DONE

Living in the moment has been blissful and liberating at times. When you're really present, you see things you never noticed before. But what about times when the moment is awful and you don't want to get more into it? The next obstacle addresses moments like those.

People are neurologically wired in such a way that memories of early trauma are triggered over and over again – until they learn to deal with them. Heart patients are prone to keep repeating the same mistakes because they haven't successfully dealt with their psychological wounds. They prefer not to talk about their past experiences. "What's done is done," and "We can't live in the past." Heart patients who lock all doors to the past continue to be influenced by the painful memories they attempt to keep out of reach.

The unpleasant fact that we may have grown up in a heart breaking environment, which shamed and invalidated us, is almost too much for us to admit. We may feel disloyal to our parents when we find them wanting. Almost all of my heart patients vigorously deny problems growing up, *at first*. They tell me how wonderful their parents were, and how much they were loved. How their parents were always there for them, went to their games, took them on vacation. Yes, their parents were punitive on occasion, but they always "deserved it." Some patients were told that they "needed" to be punished for their own good. "This will teach you to raise a hand to your brother," was the headline on a cartoon depicting a father spanking his son. As a matter of fact, it *does* teach you to raise a hand to your brother.

I have been told by several of my newer heart patients that they would come to counseling only if I agreed never to discuss their past. They didn't want to get into all that "Freudian bullshit." I had to walk on eggshells with these patients before I could gently explore some of the events that impacted their lives.

Only as we begin to explore our somewhat idealized version of childhood do we begin to see the harsher reality. My patients had forgotten some of the less pleasant facts, distorted others, and rationalized away many of the more difficult details of their lives. They were ashamed of their backgrounds and couldn't deal with their feelings.

When you feel invalidated as a child, the pain can be intense. When your whole being is called into question, rather than your errant behaviors, you risk psychological damage. Is it any wonder that the mind arranges to protect us from these horrible experiences by burying the traumatic memories and feelings?

Problems occur when we are reminded of buried memories. Anything that threatens to reawaken painful memories creates unbearable anxiety. Situations which emotionally intelligent people handle with minor discomfort can be simply overwhelming for heart patients. While we may intend to forget the past, our painful memories have a way of affecting us in the present.

A few years ago, I had to undergo another surgical procedure to determine the extent and location of blockages discovered during a stress test. When I got home after a harrowing day of tests, I couldn't wait to stuff my face with comfort food. On the surface, my behavior made about as much sense as lighting a cigarette to calm yourself down after being told you had lung cancer.

The anxiety and fear of facing further surgery reminded me of earlier experiences in my life which were equally frightening – my previous surgery, my father's heart surgery, the memories of my father crying out in pain, begging for morphine... My response to the current situation was exactly the same as when I was a kid – raid the refrigerator for some relief. I was able to convince myself that I was "entitled" to this comfort food after such a rough day.

I discovered another reason for my irrational behavior. I found that whenever I felt invalidated, weak, needy, deficient, or unhealthy, I became angry at myself. I must have concluded early in my life that bad things only happen to bad people.

I remember being overweight as a child and being painfully embarrassed about my appearance. I would buy shirts that were too big for me, to hide my girth. I often cut classes to hide in the boiler room in the basement rather than face teasing in class. Now, as an adult, I resist buying new clothes, despite pleas from my wife. She doesn't get that the whole idea of dressing up evokes powerful and painful memories for me. A simple thing like shopping for new clothes is like going for a root canal to me.

POSTTRAUMATIC STRESS SYNDROME (PTSS)

Combat veterans who have witnessed traumatic events, like the death of their fellow soldiers in battle, are subject to a condition called Posttraumatic Stress Syndrome (PTSS). I believe that heart patients have suffered experiences which threatened their emotional survival, in a manner comparable to the experiences of combat vets, whose physical survival is threatened.

If feelings of shame and invalidation were continuously evoked in childhood, a pathway is established in the brain, like a rut in a dirt road. Against the driver's wishes, the car tends to travel in the rut. Repeated traumatic experiences emblazon pathways in our neurological wiring, making it easier for new similar experiences to travel down that same pathway. So, if you are in a current situation which is reminiscent of a time in your childhood where you felt shamed or invalidated, you would respond with the same sense of being under attack – complete with adrenalin spill and increased blood pressure – as if you were in the heat of battle and heard a loud bang nearby.

Victims of this condition are never the same biologically. Anxiety, fear, hypervigilence, readiness for flight/fight, and secretion of stress hormones are some of the responses that follow exposure to circumstances perceived as life threatening. Stress hormones, triggered by threat, directly damage the heart by causing inflammation, building up plaque, and disrupting heart rhythms.

Did you know that combat vets diagnosed with this condition are at increased risk for heart disease? Even children can be diagnosed with this condition. In fact, 25% of foster home children suffer from Posttraumatic Stress Syndrome.

FAULTY WIRING

Impressions of traumatic or invalidating experiences are stored in the area of the brain known as the limbic system. More precisely, in an almond shaped structure near the bottom of the limbic system, called the amygdala.

The amygdala acts as a neural tripwire, sending out emergency calls whenever it perceives danger. Secretions of flight/flight hormones, cardiovascular reactivity, and mobilization of the movement and action centers in the body, all accompany the perception of trouble.

According to Daniel Goleman, a pioneer in Emotional Intelligence, the problem is that this alarm system is very sloppy and imprecise. It sends out urgent messages based on a crude matching system. The present circumstance need be only vaguely similar to the traumatic memories already stored, to trigger a full blown amygdala storm. It may respond as if you are in a dangerous situation when the current situation is not dangerous at all.

JOURNAL REFLECTION – STEP 7

Do you frequently overreact to situations? Which ones? Do you know why?
Do you often dwell on the past, or hope for a better future?
What are you doing when you lose track of time – when you are "in the flow"?

STEP 8 – LET LOVE IN

Choose emotional intimacy over loneliness and isolation.

When you try to figure out what went wrong in your life, you may be tempted to ask, "Why couldn't my parents have been evolved and caring? Why weren't they capable of expressing abundant love to me?" "Why did they have to be so _____?" (In truth, your parents were hurt and wounded, just as you were.) For whatever reasons, you didn't get what you wanted from them, and you're still feeling that void. Other hurts hang over from childhood. You may think back and ask, "Why wouldn't they listen to me?" "Why didn't we ever get to do what I wanted?" You felt invalidated. You're still struggling with feeling invalidated.

For you to be free to live a healthy lifestyle, you need to make peace with your laments. One way for you to make progress with this is to consider the counterpoints to your issues. After all, you're here. You are not a basket case. OK, you have problems but you're not a bad person. There are some things you love in your life.

There is a much more powerful way to heal these psychological scars. Simply allow yourself to imagine the feelings you wish you had. Consider having felt invalidated by your parents. How could they have "proven" to you that they really did take you seriously and treat you with respect? What could they have said or done that you would have taken for "proof" that they valued you?

Picture it vividly; include their voices and even their mannerisms. When you have envisioned the scene and their actions, or figured out the perfect words they would say, hold onto that image. Continue to hold onto it. Put it somewhere in your mind where you can access it easily. Take it out and replay it – often. Visualization is a wonderful tool. It can be used to heal negative energies and help you accept the way things were and are. Use it liberally to ease your mind.

Hurtful things happened to you. You can't change that. But you can change the way you hold the memories of that pain. You can find a way to accept those memories that doesn't cost you so much. You can stop letting them rob you of your aliveness. You start to heal when you accept that things did happen that hurt you. The next time that memory comes up for review, there's not so much painfully charged energy associated with it. Eventually, even the most awful memories can be looked upon without acute discomfort.

There are people who have hurt you, purposely or inadvertently. Start with your parents. Nobody gets through childhood unscathed. Even you have hurt yourself with self-doubt and shame. But you don't have to continue to do so. You can forgive. When you forgive, the hurt becomes less potent. Start by forgiving yourself. You did what you did. It was wrong and hurtful. If you could undo it, you would. You are human and you made mistakes. Forgive yourself and know that you are committed to healing yourself.

The most important reason to clear your mind of emotional pain from your past is to make room for the beautiful feelings that are available to you. The best of these is love. Chances are, people have tried to love you but you distanced them. That's what most heart patients do. But now you're less guarded, more willing to be vulnerable. You are willing to consider yourself lovable and to let the love in.

You are lovable. We all are. Some of us make it less obvious. When you begin to hold that you are a worthwhile individual (who has made mistakes and learned from them) you begin to feel worthy of receiving love. Intimacy is among the most rewarding emotions a human being can experience. It can anchor you in your quest for health.

MY PERSONAL STEP 8

I often wondered why I was only a little motivated to give up my unhealthy habits. Whenever my daughter told me that she loved me, or that she was afraid I might not be around to hug my grandchild, why didn't that alter my behavior for good? Similarly, it was curious that no matter how many times my wife told me that she needed me, or how she would be lost without me, or how my son and daughter would be devastated if I weren't around, I couldn't really let her messages of love reach me or motivate me to change. There seemed to be a part of me that was afraid to let the love in, afraid to feel vulnerable and needy. I wasn't about to let down my guard.

I realize now that I must have felt unlovable deep down inside. Growing up in an invalidating environment had had a profound effect on me. It's hard to feel lovable, when you are frequently shamed and invalidated as a child. Yet, it is vital for our survival that we learn to let the messages of love reach us.

To let the love in I had to learn to love myself. We can't trust that others can love us until we find something loveable within first. This means that we have to love the parts of ourselves that we have rejected or disowned as children. We rejected parts of ourselves that couldn't be tolerated by our parents.

To let the love in I learned that I have to accept all of my experiences, just as they are. To do this well, I have to identify my feelings at the moment and not push them away. For example, saying to myself, "I shouldn't be feeling this way," is resisting and avoiding what I am feeling at the moment. This denies my present reality and dishonors me. Let whatever is, be. When I allow my experiences full expression, I get to know and value more of myself. I set the stage for new learning as I discover aspects of myself that I may or may not want to change.

FEAR OF FINDING OUT

When you have doubts as to whether or not you are truly loveable, there is a part of you that is afraid to find out. You put some emotional distance between yourself and others, or you force them to jump through hoops until you finally trust them enough to let love in. Protecting yourself from possible rejection is not worth the price you pay.

The price you pay is that you remain stuck with your suspicion that you are unlovable. You never give yourself a chance to find out how loveable you really are. You never really heal your wounds; you are a sitting duck waiting for the next thing to trigger you. You are vulnerable to the unhealthy behaviors you use to quash painful feelings. In effect, you are waiting to prove to yourself that you were right all along – that you are unlovable.

WHY IT'S HARD TO LET THE LOVE IN

If your parents told that your needs were excessive or inappropriate, or that your character traits were unacceptable, you would begin to dislike, even hate yourself. You come to dislike everything about yourself that was unacceptable to your parents. This can include your needs, your sexuality, your appearance, your feelings, your vulnerabilities, and character traits such as timidity or aggressiveness. It is because we have self hatred that we don't feel loveable.

It is very hard for people to see that self hatred may be driving them. It seems too strong a statement to be true. Yet many people are filled with self criticism and self doubt which signals that there is at least some degree of dislike or dissatisfaction of the self in them. If you find yourself constantly busy doing things or are preoccupied with getting things done, there is a good chance that you are distracting yourself. What are you distracting yourself from? You may be distracting yourself from simply being with yourself. It is possible that you just don't like yourself very much.

How could it be otherwise? You concluded that something is "wrong" with you the way you are. You have to be someone other than yourself just to have a chance of being loved. This means you have to watch yourself carefully and hide a good deal of yourself lest others find you unacceptable. Your experience in life is one of caution and reserve.

I have noticed that at social situations my wife is usually surrounded by others and fully engaged in conversation with them. She is what I would describe as fully present. She is in her experience in the moment. I, on the other hand, am usually off in a corner of the room talking to one individual about nothing, watching myself in conversation, wondering how I'm coming across. Not only does this behavior lack spontaneity and authenticity, there is no way for intimacy to develop while I am busy defending myself.

It would be better for me to acknowledge (at least to myself) that I am fearful of rejection. I could then talk to myself about my fears and calm myself down. Perhaps I could disclose that social gatherings made me uncomfortable because I felt that I couldn't be myself. By accepting my experience in that moment, I would be practicing a form of self love – self acceptance. I can choose to accept the feelings I feel in the present; I do not need to resist the pain as I did when I was a child.

To overcome self hatred and to let the love in, you must have compassion for yourself and your feelings. It is important that you recognize that you did the best you could do in a difficult situation. Your parents, because of their own troubles and circumstances, were unable to validate important aspects of your personality.

It was difficult for either one of my parents to deal with my sister and me whenever we had needs for attention, approval, or affection, since my father was frequently sick in bed and my mother worked long hours to support the family. I would be sent to my room at the first hint of being upset with my circumstances. There was really no place in my household for a child with needs, because both parents were operating beyond capacity just to make ends meet. In order to survive in this environment, I had to buy into my parents' perceptions that I needed too much, or risk a worse fate, namely, that the parents who I depended upon for survival, might abandon me because I was a "complainer" or "unappreciative."

Once a child has concluded that he is not loved, it is not much of a stretch to conclude that he is unlovable. Following that, he doesn't believe that people really *can* love him, even when they proclaim to. When my wife tells me that she loves me, her words stand in sharp contrast to my painful early messages that my needs for more attention, affection, approval, and love are invalid.

This is pain that I try to avoid by dismissing my wife's declarations of love, as "just some things married people say to each other to keep things flowing smoothly." Of course, this leaves my parents' negative messages intact. Old messages take precedence over new ones that are trying to get through – the old messages have been with me much longer. My old messages have become the reality against which new messages are evaluated and frequently dismissed.

HOW TO GET THE LOVE YOU NEED

Having felt victimized by life, heart patients may feel entitled to some restitution. Their focus is often on "What's in it for me?" and "What can I get from this relationship or circumstance?"

Many people operate on a barter system. We expect something in return for our giving, be it money, love, appreciation or admiration. The problem with this barter system is that we often think are not getting enough back for what we are putting out. This leads us down the path of manipulation and control, to make sure that we don't get conned or short changed, so that we don't feel used or taken advantage of. It also opens the door to anger when we do feel short changed or conned (and we often do). Another problem is that we never get enough to feel satisfied. No matter how much love, praise, or money we get, we always want more. Worse, we have to hold on to what we have for dear life, afraid that it might be taken away somehow.

Bartering is exactly the wrong formula for getting what you need. What you need is the feeling of abundance or satisfaction that you never had as a child growing up in an environment of scarcity and deprivation.

Here's the rub. According to Susan Jeffers, author of *Feel the Fear and Do It Anyway*, "It's easy to give when you are feeling abundantly endowed, but you only feel that way when you give, not before." In other words, it is giving that gives you the feeling of abundance. How strange is that!? Heart patients are in the habit of feeling depleted when they give. Or they give with the expectation of getting. This is because we are constantly aware of a set of scales which tips in the wrong direction when we give, and tips in our favor when we get. We need to practice giving in order to see the paradox that the more we give, the more of us there is to give.

The key is to focus on what you can give instead of what you can get. According to Susan Jeffers, "If your purpose in life is to give, you can't be conned. This is because if someone takes they are simply fulfilling your life's purpose."

People may give to you out of guilt or fear or a desire to get back from you what they are giving. These gifts are a poor substitute for gifts of love spontaneously generated from the heart. Many patients don't know the difference or seem to care.

We are so intent on getting, that for us, even coerced receiving is better than none at all.

You can change the quality of the gifts you receive by shifting your focus to giving. What goes around comes around. This can be as simple as giving acknowledgment. Just by telling a person what difference they made in your life you contribute to that person's well being. Listening is another way of making a contribution. Warm and tender responses may greet you when you give others the gift of your attentive listening.

Too often, we are so busy with "important stuff" that we neglect those people who most need us (the ones we most need). In truth, it is easier for many of us to attend to tasks than it is to be with others. For example, some of my heart patients would often prefer to stay late at work (for the "good" of the family), rather than spend time with their kids. What they miss out on is the closeness with family that can be a refuge – a source of intimacy which is healing. They also forfeit a cache of memories from which to draw pride and inspiration.

When you think about a moment in your life that you truly cherished, chances are that your memory involved other people. Most likely, the people in your fondest memories were filled with life. Maybe you thought about your daughter's wedding, or your spouse's face upon holding your child for the first time. Maybe you were watching your kids frolic in the ocean. What made these moments special was the sheer aliveness and joy that you participated in or were witness to.

The greatest gift you can give someone is the experience of a truly alive and exuberant you. This may be a far cry from where you see yourself at this moment. But take heart, you gain a degree of spontaneity and vitality as your energy returns. People want to be with you when you are feeling good about yourself and are engaged in healthy activities. They want to share in your aliveness and enthusiasm. Your greatest gift to others is a healthy and vital you. Be that gift!

OBSTACLE 8: KEEP YOUR ACT TOGETHER

> *You are loved. You know you are. But every now and then a thought creeps in to spoil that beautiful feeling. What if they knew who I really was? Would they love me if I didn't act the way I do? This is an obstacle in your path to true health. Treat it as you have the other obstacles up to this point. Recognize it, go around it, and carry on with your valuable journey.*

Heart patients often wear masks while living out their lives. They show themselves to be tough and in control, or kind and caring, all the while covering feelings of shame and inadequacy. In order to live authentically, they must resolve these feelings and remove their masks.

MASKS

Some masks are obvious. People wear obvious masks around Halloween. Everyone knows that you are only pretending to be Batman or The Lone Ranger. Kids love to put on these kinds of masks. Most of us symbolically put on this kind of mask when we pretend to have special powers. I joke with my seventeen year old son about my rock hard stomach and superhuman intelligence. Wearing a mask like this is no more than harmless play; it is not dangerous to health.

In contrast, people may wear "hidden" masks. Masks are put between you and the real world to conceal your image. Like sunglasses they filter unwanted reality and create blind spots. By disowning or denying prominent personality traits, hidden masks keep your act together at the expense of your health.

When you are wearing a hidden mask, others may sense that there is discordance between what you say and your behavior. You may state that you are open to new ideas, but your co-workers and friends may be full of bullet holes. You can wear a mask for so long that you are no longer aware that you have it on. This is especially true when masks are donned very early in life.

You can dress up like a king for Halloween, compete with crown, robe, and scepter. Everyone (including you) knows that you are pretending to be a king. But what if you didn't know it was an act? You might feel entitled to special treatment. You may require admiration, behave in a haughty manner, and manipulate others (for their own good).

There is no way you can tell that you are wearing a mask by looking within. The only way that you can find out if you are wearing a mask is by monitoring your circumstances. If you've been married seven times, it may dawn on you that you have a problem with intimacy and are masking it. If you don't have many friends, there's a good chance that you are not being authentic, masking your true colors. When you finally realize that you are wearing a mask, you can take it off. When you take off your mask, you become open to authentic self expression. People will relate to you more intimately because what they see is what they get.

HIDING YOUR FEELINGS IS BAD FOR YOUR HEALTH

No one would advocate the practice of making every feeling public. Marriages would not survive if every spouse responded truthfully to such questions as, "Do I look good in this?" However, habitually keeping feelings inside, particularly negative feelings, can be damaging to your health.

Our fear of revealing who we really are or how we truly feel, effects health negatively in a variety of ways:

- Any fear subjects the body to a flood of stress hormones. Fear of exposing your true self leaves you vulnerable to this bombardment.
- When you are afraid to be yourself, a good deal of energy is spent trying to appear other than you are. It takes exertion to hold up a mask or a false front to others.
- Feelings that are not dealt with properly often lead to behaviors that are not healthy.
- If you mask your depression, and don't adequately recognize or handle this negative feeling, you tend to withdraw from others. Studies have shown that depression increases the chance of a heart attack by more than fourfold.
- If you mask your anger, and don't acknowledge it to yourself or others, you cannot discharge it appropriately. You may become too explosive. Studies

have found that undischarged anger can increase blood pressure and release damaging stress hormones.

- Hiding who you are deprives you of the healing powers of close relationships. By keeping your true feelings to yourself, you deprive yourself of the experience of being loved deeply and unconditionally.

Research has demonstrated conclusively that intimacy is particularly beneficial for heart patients. Mortality was significantly higher for heart patients who had no one to confide in. And feelings of being loved and emotionally supported were found to be more important predictors of the severity of blockages than are hypertension, smoking, cholesterol and other risk factors.

THE OPEN PERSONALITY

Research conducted with people who have survived the most adverse of circumstances, such as war time paratroopers or concentration camp survivors, reveals two common characteristics.

First is the importance of their values to their personality. Values provide direction; they are a source of continuity and stability during extremely stressful times. Victor Frankl, author of *Man's Search for Meaning*, found that many of his fellow concentration camp survivors were made stronger by adversity because the extreme conditions forced them to clarify their values.

A second characteristic common to these survivors is that they were able to draw upon a wide range of emotions and personality traits. This ability made them more adaptive in social situations and enabled them to develop life saving support systems under extreme conditions. For example, they were tough in dealing with the harsh prison conditions but tender in dealing with fellow prisoners who were wounded. Al Seibert, author of *The Survivor Personality* and a former paratrooper, found that the most prominent feature of survivors was the paradoxical nature of their personalities.

Survivors' personalities are made up of opposite personality traits. Paradoxically, they can be serious and playful, generous and selfish, logical and intuitive, powerful and vulnerable, rigid and flexible. To have access to opposite sides of the personality is an extremely adaptive emotional capacity. A personality that tolerates opposites within itself, is more tolerant of others, less defensive, more flexible, and ultimately, healthier than a personality composed of a narrower range of traits. The more diversity and variety existing within a system, the greater the ability to cope outside the system.

The mind of a healthy and powerful person is spacious, having ample room for conflicting feelings, contradictory ideas, and life's paradoxes. It may be easier to understand this concept if you think about something more concrete, like painting a picture. If you want to paint, is yellow the only color on your palette? Or do you want to use blue as well? (They are opposite from one another on a color wheel.) In daily life having a fuller palette of emotional responses to draw upon makes us better able to weather emotional storms.

In contrast to an open personality, people with "avoidant" personalities tend to disown or deny certain aspects of their personality. The banishment of large parts of their personality, leaves them with fewer resources to deal with stress, and makes them less adaptive to change. The avoidant person will be more likely to demonstrate only one side of paradoxical personality traits. He will be rigid instead of rigid *and* flexible, logical instead of logical *and* intuitive, tough instead of tough *and* tender.

One dimensional individuals may pride themselves on being consistent. More accurately, they are unaware that very valuable segments of their personalities are simply unavailable to them. Individuals with personalities classified primarily as rigid, pessimistic, defensive, serious, or non-expressive, were found to be at risk for heart disease.

Heart patients are likely to have submerged the trusting aspects of their personalities in favor of their suspicious aspects. If they have been on the receiving end of too many broken promises, this is a predictable result. If they were the ones who broke promises, they come to distrust themselves. If you repeatedly break your commitments to live a healthy lifestyle you will be suspicious and distrustful of your own word.

Wouldn't it be wonderful if you could keep your ability to discern real threat (distrust) and balance it with trust, giving others the benefit of the doubt? Could you do the same with yourself? You are at the point where you can choose to trust yourself. You've earned trust just by getting this far in the book. You can follow through on your intentions.

JOURNAL REFLECTION – STEP 8

Can you share your deepest feelings with someone? Who?
What weren't you allowed to express as a child?
What masks do you wear?

STEP 9 – CREATE A NEW MISSION

Who you are is who you need to be to live life to the fullest. How does that look to you? What would you do if you could do anything? This kind of thinking leads to the next and final step. Congratulations. You have given yourself a surprise gift. What will it be? Take this final step and discover your gift.

Design the rest of your life.

Most of us have a story or life script which can be encapsulated in a few paragraphs. My original story would appear as follows:

I was raised in a working class suburb, the son of a disabled war veteran who was always sick. He was in and out of hospitals and we were scared to death he wouldn't make it. But when he was home, my father was a tyrant. He lashed out at us and we were terrified. We had very little money, and only one can of soup had to feed four faces. We were desperate. The neighbors helped to raise me and felt sorry for me. Once the neighbors chipped in and sent me to summer camp for underprivileged children. The family overcame great odds. My father eventually went to college late in life, despite being 100% disabled, according to Uncle Sam. We were proud of him. We eventually relocated to a better neighborhood. Although my father was harsh and abusive because of his illness, he later softened up. My mother was a "saint" for putting up with such hardships.

Versions of this story of my life have been repeated hundreds of times to anyone who would listen. It seemed very real to me, just as my beliefs seemed like facts to me. The story is perhaps unconsciously designed to elicit sympathy, but also tells the listener that I am from a family of fighters, and by extension, I am a force to be reckoned with.

The problems with this narrative of my life (and any narrative) are that, first, it can define my life and, second, the story is untrue. My life became an extension of the drama that I envisioned, not the reality of what actually happened.

Exercise: Rewrite your story from the point of view of reality, taking all the drama and interpretations out of it. Just stick to the facts. If you have any experience with a navigation system in a car, you would recognize the navigator's voice as being dispassionate and factual. "She" doesn't get upset with you for making a wrong turn. Nor does she panic. She just calls it like it is, without elaboration or emotion. Try to rewrite your story in the navigator's voice. For example, to take the drama out of my story, I would rewrite it the following way:

> I am the son of a father who was ill. I have a sister. When he was not in the hospital, my father was frequently angry. We lived in a neighborhood with lots of kids and neighbors. My grandmother and aunt lived with us for several years. The family lived on income from the government, supplemented by my grandmother's rent and my mother's job. The neighbors would occasionally help out my family. Later, as my father began to recover, he went to college. He became a psychologist. We relocated to a larger house. My father became more approachable. My mother supported the family in many ways.

This rewritten story captures more of the reality of the situation, rather than the drama, from which my identity took shape (King Larry). It would be hard to derive a Poor Larry identity from my story devoid of interpretation and drama.

You are not your story. Your story happened. End of story. Not end of you! Consider this to be the beginning of your story – Part II: My Journey to a Healthy lifestyle. Design the next few chapters. Where do you see yourself tomorrow, -next month, -three years from now? Envision yourself living the life you want, by wise design and choice.

You have everything you need to live your life with integrity and self-esteem – you have yourself. Look deep within yourself to find your core values. You are the source of all your thoughts, visions, and inspiration. Consider your dearest desires when you make decisions and choices. Let your actions spring from the sincere desire to live a healthy life – physically and emotionally. Let this begin a brand new era in your life – one with a healthy ending.

MY PERSONAL STEP 9

I learned firsthand that the process of looking deeply into ourselves, though difficult, results in the discovery of a more powerful person. We learn to love ourselves, let others love us, and become more of who we can be.

I am now 65 years old. I have a wonderful wife, two great kids and two grandchildren. I run a five mile race every year and walk four miles a day to stay in shape. I play a mean set of doubles and just made my first bogie in golf. Recently, I beat a group of teenagers, which included my six-foot-four son, in a pick-up basketball game (I had more than a little help from my friends). I continue to counsel patients, give lectures and workshops, and write. I am blessed with good friends, and have discovered meaning in my life on a daily basis.

HOW TO DISCOVER YOUR VALUES

It is difficult to find your deepest values by yourself. You may need your spouse or friends to help you. This is because you have been so busy living your life that you have never stopped to look at it. One day my patient, Sam, admitted to me, "You know, I haven't a clue as to who I really am. I've followed what I was supposed to do my whole life and I don't even know if I'm happy about how my life turned out."

Here are three questions that Lee Eisenberg used in his book, *The Number,* to help people discover what they valued:

- If you suddenly came into enough money to live comfortably for the rest of your life, what would you do differently?
- If your doctor discovered a rare illness and gave you five to six years to live, how would you live your life?
- What if the doctor gave you the really bad news that you have 24 hours to live? What would you miss? Who did you not get to be? What did you not do that you wanted to do?

We might as well finish you off now that we have taken your health from bad to worse! So next, I would like you to imagine your own funeral. Your friends and loved ones have met to celebrate your life. Who would be there and what would they be saying about you? For what qualities would you be remembered? Does this please you? Did you make a difference in the lives of those attending? If so, how?

Finally, there are a few other important questions that you can ask to round out your search for deeper understanding of what you most value:

- What are the qualities of character that you most admire in others?
- What do you enjoy doing when you have nothing pressing to do?
- What are you doing when you lose track of time?
- What is so important in your life that you would be willing to die for it?
- Who are the people in history you most admire, and why?
- Who is living the life that you most envy? Why?

- What have been your moments of greatest satisfaction, and what do they have in common?
- What would you do if you had more courage?

DRAFTING YOUR MISSION STATEMENT

It is time to incorporate what you learned about yourself into a mission statement which is often only a single sentence long. Your mission statement includes who you would like to be, what you would like to do, and the values you choose to live by. Done well, your mission statement can reinvigorate you and give you a new lease on life.

Start by picking some action words that are meaningful and exciting to you. I am grateful to my friend, Susanne Sweeny, author of *Transform Stress into Strength*, for her insights here. Action words include: accomplish, acquire, advance, affirm, alleviate, appear, communicate, compel, create, demonstrate, distribute, drive, embolden, empower, enable, educate, embrace, engage, engineer, foster, facilitate, help, launch, lead, mentor, model, motivate, nurture, persuade, produce, promote, reform, restore, safeguard, serve, sustain, touch, utilize, validate, venture, volunteer.

Next, list some of the values that you have discovered about yourself, which will serve as guideposts for the rest of your life. Examples here would include: justice, family, teaching, freedom, fair play, reliability, honesty, consistency, responsibility, service, dependability, integrity, authenticity, excellence, creativity.

Last, ask yourself who you are here to help. Examples are: environment, healthcare, home owners, children, the poor, agriculture, heart patients, nutrition, law, politics, government, civil rights issues, disabled, women's issues, gardening.

Now you are ready to come up with your own mission statement, which would look something like this:

> My mission is to _____, _____, and _____ *(your three action words)* _____ *(group or cause that excites you)*, to, for or with _____ *(your core values or purpose)*.

My own personal mission statement is: "My mission is to mentor, embolden, and empower people to sustain the lifestyle changes necessary for their well-being."

This mission statement stands in stark contrast to what King Larry would have written: "My mission is to use my professional position to help others, to make myself appear intelligent, and to accumulate wealth, power and prestige."

King Larry's mission statement was based upon myths that I accepted as true. My current mission statement is based upon what I discovered about my true self.

Research shows that people who use their strengths for purposes larger than themselves experience more of a sense of purpose and meaning in their lives. A new mission in life is more than a change in what you do. It is a change in who you are. Freud said, "The child is father to the man." What he meant was that our experiences in childhood determine what kind of adults we become. People on a mission see things from a different perspective. Instead of being pushed into the future by past experiences or beliefs, a person with a new mission has invented his future.

Will you choose to remain on the same trajectory dictated by your past experiences and beliefs (as Freud predicted) or can you allow yourself to be impelled forward by your new mission? This book was a vision that gave my present life meaning and direction.

What does all this mean to a practically-minded person such as you? Bottom line: You have a better chance of sticking to lifestyle changes when you change who you are. It makes changing what you do that much easier and more natural. You are not a loser in life's lottery, or a victim of your invalidating experiences. Instead you are a champion of your own making.

JOURNAL REFLECTION – STEP 9

As the *one in ten,*, what new behaviors will support your heart healthy lifestyle?

THE TRANSFORMED YOU

You are now in a position to go a step beyond change. You are ready to take a step of transformation.

Transformation is not just the acquisition of more information or a better way of doing things. It is a shift in who you are being. When you see the world through a new set of lenses, you have transformed the way in which information comes into you and is processed by you. You don't see people in the same way and obstacles tend to disappear. People who have transformed themselves describe it as going beyond their self imposed limits. They no longer feel trapped in their minds.

A transformed individual steps out of himself and considers his life from a new perspective. He perceives himself, his world, and time in a new way. The transformed person is not pushed into the future by emotional wounds. He has looked at and resolved his painful experiences from the past. Instead, he invents a future that provides his present moment with purpose and direction. The past remains only a dim, probably inaccurate, memory of what happened. It no longer has the power to dictate his future.

For people addicted to unhealthy lifestyles, transformation is the key to recovery. In the course of transformation, emotions are recognized and appropriately expressed. Energy that was bound in self defense is freed up; it is freed up to make healthy choices. You become the *one in ten* who sustains a heart healthy lifestyle.

AFTERWORD

The day before my father died he called me into his hospital room. He wanted to share some final thoughts and feelings with me. With tears in his eyes, my father told me that he loved me. He was crying as he apologized for not telling me this often enough in my life. He said that he was proud of me and that I was a good son. I watched as my father transformed himself before my eyes. At that moment he revealed a side of himself that I had only caught glimpses of before. His heartfelt feelings touched me deeply. I never felt such a deep understanding of who my father was, and such love for him at that moment.

We heart patients are tough customers, and this book has not been easy for me to write or you to read. I am convinced however, that despite our thick skins and rigid beliefs, we have the desire to experience ourselves at our best, to realize our fullest potential and to be all that is possible for us. We know intuitively the difference between a mission that has heart, and a blind walk on a well trodden path. And we don't have to wait until our last days on earth to begin the journey. By getting through this book, you have demonstrated courage in the face of uncertainty, a willingness to keep an open mind, and at the deepest level, the ability to risk your own life. You have opened yourself to a way of being which gives you real control of how your life turns out. You have your hands on the steering wheel instead of on the rear view mirror.

You and I have embarked on a journey of truth, much as my father did. This book has helped me, and I hope you as well, to look deeply inside ourselves for the source of our suffering and the seeds of our recovery. We have tremendous power within us to create ourselves anew. When we discover this power, we realize that disease is not a death sentence. Rather it is an opportunity to heal very deep emotional hurts to our hearts. By becoming true to ourselves, we can experience the joy and aliveness that has been too long suppressed by the hard hearted sides of our personalities. Everything is possible when we soften our hearts. We become fearless in the face of uncertainty or criticism. And our lives become full of curiosity, enchantment, and magic.

CASE HISTORIES

BERNIE

It was the fall of 1998 and Bernie had recently moved his three year old Consulting practice into his home. The move would allow him to care for his three month old son, work part-time, lower his expenses and be a stay at home dad. His wife, who was a teacher, had just returned to work full-time. Bernie was at his desk paying bills, when he became completely over whelmed with anger. There wasn't enough money to pay the bills, his business was almost non-existent and his family life was in turmoil – sleep deprivation, unpredictable schedules, and holidays approaching.

He felt like a failure. He remembers putting his head down and saying to himself "something has to give." Less than a week later, Bernie experienced three increasingly more painful episodes of chest pain. He casually asked his wife one evening – "What does a Gall Bladder Attack feel like? (Someone once told him that a Gall bladder attack can cause chest pain. Bernie sensed there was a problem with his heart, but was in denial.)

He ended up in his doctor's office the next morning and was sent directly to the emergency room. He was given medication and scheduled for a catheterization. The doctors were not able to unblock his arteries. Bernie underwent triple bypass surgery later that day. He was only 39 years old. He had a 5 year old son and a three month old son.

After surgery, it was recommended that Bernie participate in a Cardiac Rehab Program. He started the program three months after surgery and began exercising 3 times a week, learned about diet, life style and medications. "I began to incorporate all of these things into my life. However, I was still scared to death and felt alone", Bernie said. During one of the education classes at Cardiac Rehab, a discussion about psychological factors (feelings of anger, depression, not feeling loved) and behaviors (impulsiveness, denial, entitlement) and Type A personalities prompted Bernie to ask himself, "could this be me?"

He started to realize that there may be more to heart disease than genetics and high cholesterol. This gave him some hope that he could do something about his health, rather than bemoan his genetic predisposition towards heart disease. He spoke with one of the Rehab Nurses who referred him to my office.

Throughout his life, Bernie struggled with anger, frustration, low self esteem, feelings of entitlement and general feelings of "not fitting in" and "being different". Our first order of business was to uncover the invalidating circumstances responsible for these feelings.

Bernie grew up in a two parent family with a twin sister. His parents had a difficult time having children so the children were considered a "blessing" when they arrived. Neither parent was college educated. And both parents grew up during the depression. Bernie's father worked various sales and service jobs. His mother was a stay at home mom until the children went to high school. His parents were able to provide the basic necessities but no extras. Money was never discussed but Bernie knew there were problems at times.

Bernie's father died at age 51 from an accident. Bernie was devastated upon the death of his father. "How could God do this to me? I was still a young man who needed his father," Bernie lamented.

Bernie always felt that his parents, particularly his mother, were "over – protective." He wasn't allowed to play little league baseball because "the coaches yelled at the players." He was prohibited from being with his friends, because "I had to cross a busy street." At age 17, Bernie wasn't allowed to go to college away from home, because "I might start selling drugs, like my cousin." Bernie always felt he had to be good. "I wasn't permitted nor would I let myself do anything bad. I was mister goody two shoes," says Bernie.

Bernie felt very weak and insecure and was shy around strangers and later around girls. Throughout college and his early twenties, Bernie never had a relationship with a woman that lasted more than 6 months. He was always too "sensitive" and was often told that he was an "angry young man." "I felt like people didn't like me, I wasn't good looking enough or cool enough," said Bernie. "I placed a lot of value on how others viewed me. I really did not like myself." It was obvious that Bernie needed to get a better handle on his emotions. He took things too personally and reacted with anger whenever things didn't work out like they should ("should" as defined by Bernie).

By overprotecting Bernie, his parents inadvertently invalidated him. His self confidence was diminished. The second goal for Bernie was to repair the damaged self esteem which resulted from these invalidating experiences. Just providing a sympathetic ear was enough for Bernie to begin to feel validated. Encouraging him to try out new things in his business reinforced a sense of initiative and potency and resulted in establishing a beautiful new office (outside his home) which was an immediate boost for his ego and his professional status. After narrowly missing a cutoff score on a difficult test he was hoping would further his career, Bernie was encouraged to try again. This time he passed an important consulting course which elevated his status in the company. This resolve was used to help Bernie see that he was not a prisoner of his genes and that he could make the lifestyle changes which could extend his life.

When we first met for individual therapy I asked Bernie to read my book, *A Change of Heart*. His reaction to the book was interesting. "I thought how ironic. Here is a guy who thinks he is an expert on heart disease because he has written a book. Must be some great advice, after all it didn't work for him. What was I going to learn that I didn't already know? I just wanted to join the support group, not be psychoanalyzed by this guy." "I was a little arrogant and angry," Bernie recalled. He was also quite suspicious and distrustful, like most of my heart patients who come for help.

One day while reading my book, Bernie came across a statement/ question that set off a light bulb. "Was he a human doing or a human being?" This was it for Bernie. He found what he had been searching for. He was a human doing, not a human being! "I wasn't living life; I was existing to take care of others, pleasing everyone around me, always doing the right thing! Not talking about my pain, emotions or feelings! All this time I though I was doing the best I could do but what I really was doing was neglecting the most important person, ME! Always doing and never being!" He had bought into the myth that you are only valued for what you produce, not who you are.

Bernie learned to change his "should" thinking to "I want to" thinking. He learned to listen to his self talk and not let it overwhelm him with negative thoughts. He learned to accept that he was not perfect and that it is ok to make a mistake. He learned to be self forgiving and forgiving of others. "I respect myself now, and like the person I am," says Bernie.

Bernie also saw that he was not the entitled person (king) that he thought he was. He saw that his arrogant behavior was just a cover-up for feelings of low self esteem. He discovered that, "If I work hard, am honest with myself and others, recognize my limitations and my short comings, accept responsibility for my behaviors, acknowledge and let go of my past hurt, I will get the love and respect from others that I have always craved," he now believes. He has developed humility in the best sense of the word.

In the past Bernie used to give with the expectation that he would get the recognition he deserved. Today, he gives to others for the feeling it gives him in being able and fortunate enough to help someone in need. He became a volunteer in a unique hospital program designed to assist heart patients. Meanwhile, and not incidentally, his business has been flourishing.

Bernie is a changed person. He can openly acknowledge his mistakes and take responsibility for his behaviors. He has learned to control his anger and negative thoughts through expressing his feelings, exercising regularly, following a healthy diet, taking medication as prescribed and forgiving himself and others when necessary. He has learned to make choices for himself and not others. "I choose to do things because I want to, not because I should," says Bernie. He realized that he was on a path of self destruction and did not want to expose his family to the premature death of a father and husband. Realizing this motivated him to sustain the changes he embarked upon.

"December 7th, 1998 was my rebirth. I am not perfect and have a lot of work to do, but I feel and truly believe that today, I have the tools, knowledge and understanding to live to see my grandchildren and live a long and healthy life."

MARY

Mary struggled with cancer and heart disease. She had heart surgery six years before she was referred to my office. Mary was experiencing serious marital problems and felt unsupported by her husband particularly with respect to her medical condition. There was very little communication between them, and they had not had sexual relations in years. This was Mary's second marriage. Mary's first husband, Ron, became addicted to drugs, was abusive and had difficulties holding down a job. They were married less than two years, when Mary came home from work one day to find that Ron had abandoned her without warning for another woman. Mary was angry and destroyed all evidence of her relationship with Ron. She felt humiliated and her self worth sunk to new lows. She blamed herself for the marital problems and for not being able to make Ron happy. She longed to find someone who could love her for who she was.

She met Thomas very soon after Ron left her. They married quickly and Mary thought she found the perfect husband. He appeared to be steady and dependable, and the couple was happy for a short time. Mary quickly got pregnant, and other children followed. Her husband began to feel that that he was not a priority in Mary's life. He began to withdraw from her and starting to drink heavily. Mary felt that she couldn't make Tom happy, no matter how much she catered to him. She would "try, and try again" to make him happy. The harder she tried, the more he seemed to withdraw. Thomas mostly ignored her. If Mary tried to speak up he often criticized her or trivialized her feelings. Thomas stopped having sex with Mary after their third child was born. Although Mary was an attractive and intelligent woman, Thomas told her that she was unattractive and was not stimulating to him. She felt worthless.

Mary stayed married to Thomas for 25 years. During that time she learned to "put on a happy face," and to keep her feelings to herself. She became so good at hiding her feelings that she almost didn't allow herself to feel anything at all. Mary's philosophy was "You have to do what you have to do to get things done." There was really no time or tolerance for feelings. She lived an "avoidant" lifestyle – hiding her pain from herself and others.

Mary was surprised as counseling sessions wore on that she was beginning to feel feelings that she had not experienced before. She was beginning to feel depressed. She had never felt depressed before because she considered herself to be "tough". She was able to continue her façade of toughness until her health started to suffer. In addition to her heart disease, Mary had been diagnosed with a form of cancer. At the time of her first office visit, Mary had depleted her reserves, was running on empty and was convinced she was going to die. (She reported that her doctor also felt she was near death). She reported that there was so much tension in her life that she "would explode." She had been placed on three different blood pressure medications. Mary was pessimistic about her deteriorating condition, and was told that she would probably require additional surgical procedures.

As we explored Mary's background it became clear that she had been invalidated by her parents. Mary learned that no matter what she did it was not good enough to please her mother or get affection from her father. Her father was orphaned as a young child and never had the experience of being loved. Consequently he didn't know how to express love and was unable to demonstrate his love for Mary. He worked a lot and was away from home.

Mary's mother grew up in a large Italian family where she fought for attention. She became overly critical and controlling. Mary's mother had children late in life, and expected Mary to conform to her rules. She didn't give Mary the validation that she needed. She was extremely critical and controlling. She often ignored Mary, just wanting her to play quietly by herself. She kept Mary in her crib until she was five years old. Later, Mary would play for hours in a large closet where she felt safe from ridicule. If she didn't conform to the rules, she knew she would be beaten with a big strap by her father when he got home. She became very good at denying, rationalizing and fantasizing to help her endure the pain. Mary's mother almost died in childbirth, and Mary felt guilty about being born.

Apparently, there was no sex between Mary's parents after she was born, adding to Mary's belief that she was "bad" somehow and responsible for her parent's relationship problems. She tried to be a "good girl," get good grades in school. She found that she learned quickly and was a very good student. She made a lot of friends to fill the void she felt with her parents. She soon realized that her parents were pleased with her good grades. She found some form of validation of her worth. So she continued to work harder and harder to excel, trying to do everything she felt she "should" do, and forgetting what she really wanted. She figured that the best she could do was to be loved for the things she did rather than the special person she was.

She became a social worker and was well respected in her field. Her self esteem had been shattered and work became the only place she could feel good about herself. Only by giving to others even at her own expense could she feel whole. She was pulled in every direction by her attempts to satisfy the demands of her family, relatives, and work. Consequently, she was under enormous stress and pressure, and did not have the self regulation skills necessary to protect her heart. She allowed her anxiety and fear to keep her from growing.

Mary had to discover herself apart from the "trained personality" she had assumed. Gradually, she began to see herself as a resilient and powerful person underneath an overlay of gentility and meekness. I was able to point out many examples of her not being pushed around even by people in authority. She was arrogant and imperious in certain ways, a pussycat with teeth. Seeing this allowed her to gain self respect. She no longer saw herself as a "patsy" or victim. She learned to say, "No" when stretched too thin. She learned that she was deserving of happiness and that she needn't continue a life of self sacrifice.

Mary eventually separated and divorced Tom. She bought a modest house and a new car for herself and is currently in a very satisfying, loving relationship. She joined a health club and started exercising at least three times a week. She recognizes that her need for a certain amount of space is a good thing, and can easily talk about circumstances that may have triggered her in the past. She is less reactive to feeling criticized and more independent. She continues to get awards at work, and people marvel that she is "a new person".

Mary has not required additional heart surgery as predicted and is enjoying relatively good health. Her blood pressure is under control and her heart has been stable. Her cancer was detected early and she is currently cancer free. She is still "hooked" by painful memories but not as often and her reactions are not as severe. Mary is optimistic about her future, positive about herself and grateful that she had the opportunity to understand the deeper issues affecting her health.

BILL

Bill was a patient who experienced a traumatic childhood. He was easily triggered by unresolved issues of the past. His unhealthy behaviors were designed to soothe his pain, but resulted in long term consequences to his health. It was not until he allowed himself to share his experiences that he was able to resolve them.

I first met Bill at a presentation at a local hospital where I spoke about the psychological and emotional aspects of heart disease. At the time Bill was no stranger to hospitals, having visited the catheterization lab nine times. He had undergone procedures to install five stents and had several angioplasties. Shortly after my presentation, Bill underwent bypass surgery. He required an additional procedure within three months of his bypass. At that time in his life, Bill was more than ready to hear alternatives to what his doctor was prescribing to heal his heart. He had read several books and was quite conversant about the current points of view in medicine. In fact, I remember Bill as being as knowledgeable about his condition as anyone I had seen before.

Bill was interested in a fresh and new approach at the time. He started one-on-one counseling sessions with me and after a few visits was invited to join a group of other heart patients in a weekly session. In the group, Bill was tight lipped at first. It took several months before Bill felt comfortable sharing his experiences.

Bill and I explored various ideas as to how his heart disease might have worsened. He was admittedly a "workaholic," commuting hours each day to his place of employment, staying late, and traveling extensively. He was also grossly overweight. Social activities were limited to going out to dinner with his wife. He did not have many friends. His lifestyle could best be described as "avoidant" or "constricted." It was clear that his lifestyle was not conducive to heart health.

I asked Bill to recall an early experience that may have affected how his life turned out. His response was indicative of early childhood invalidation. "I was 2 years old and at a movie with my parents. I cried and wanted the bottle, apparently causing my father embarrassment. He ordered my mother to stop giving me the bottle from that point on. She continued, but made me hide it from my father. She taught me to fear my father, but I feared her too. She once broke a plastic guitar over my head. I was lonely, afraid of opening up to others for fear of ridicule. I ballooned to 315 pounds. I learned to keep my feelings private". It was quite logical that Bill became an engineer where he could deal with numbers more than people.

Through our discussions, Bill was helped to see how these early experiences created permanent scars in his memory. He learned how his fear of having to experience the painful feelings of rejection constricted his life and how his isolation from others may have impacted his heart. "My personality was clearly related to these painful past experiences and created stress for me as well as impacting my heart disease," said Bill. He had developed a lifestyle that was designed to avoid the resurgence of painful early feelings of rejection. His obsession with work served the function of keeping his mind off what really ailed him – self doubts, feelings of alienation and of worthlessness. His eating served the function of soothing his pain short term. His lifestyle almost killed him.

Bill learned to see that he was arrogant with respect to his intelligence. His storehouse of factual information was impressive, and he was not shy about showing off. Bill's arrogance extended to his eating habits. He believed that he could be 315 pounds and still eat like a "king." Denial and rationalization were defenses that fueled this kind of unhealthy thinking and Bill's unhealthy behaviors.

Bill learned to abdicate the throne in our group therapy sessions. This happened as he became more comfortable with other people who were willing to expose their self doubts and weaknesses. He learned to value himself as others began to value him – not so much for his intelligence as for his sincere interest in their lives. Bill became a friend to the other group members, maintaining contact with them outside the office. His life took on new meaning as he discovered ways to make a difference in the community. He immersed himself in local politics and became a positive force for change.

Bill has not had a reoccurrence of angina even though there were a few trips to the hospital with what he thought were possible heart problems. During a recent thallium stress test, his doctor did not see any blockages but recommended a catheterization to be on the safe side. "It was real interesting," said Bill, "to now find that there was no blockage at all in my arteries feeding my heart."

Bill is convinced his progress is a function of his hard work in our sessions. He has learned how to cope with stress in a much more controlled fashion. Things that used to panic Bill no longer cause such stress now. For example, Bill used to be deathly afraid of appearing in public. Although he still does not relish the attention this gives him, he dos not panic at the thought of the experience. "I now believe that it is not the case that everyone is out to get me although I quite often believed this for many years."

Bill shifted from a lifestyle of avoidance to one that allowed for him to become more accepting of himself and others. As he added additional components to his personality, he became more resilient. In addition Bill feels that his self image has improved in other ways. "I would put in over and above the required number of hours at work just to prove my worth to the company. I now see this as being counter productive because the stress caused me to end up in the hospital and out of work for some time dealing with the heart disease."

Bill finally entered the pain-acceptance-health cycle after years of making himself ill. Whereas he used to resist exposing his perceived shortcomings, Bill has learned to accept his feelings and engage others socially despite his fear.

SCIENTIFIC RATIONALE

There is scientific evidence behind my treatment and protocol. The model outlined in this book is a modification and elaboration of the "Reserve Capacity Model," as proposed by Linda Gallo and Karen A. Matthews of the University of Pittsburgh. These authors attempted to understand how early psychosocial experiences increased the risk for Coronary Heart Disease (CHD) in adults. I was interested in how these early experiences led to unhealthy lifestyles, and why it was so difficult to sustain healthy choices.

It is known that childhood socioeconomic status (SES) predicts the incidence of CHD in adulthood. Gallo and Matthews set out to determine the components within SES most likely responsible for the association between SES and CHD. They defined SES as "ones level of resources or prestige in relation to others." These researchers discovered that low SES children experienced more frequent and intense negative emotions and attitudes than children from high SES homes. They presumed that low SES individuals experienced more threatening conditions and maintained fewer resources – tangible, interpersonal and intrapersonal – for dealing with stressful events as compared with others.

My psychology practice is located in a suburb north of Philadelphia. Many of my heart disease patients grew up in affluent homes with tangible assets. Yet the majority of them could be described as having a "smaller bank of resources" when faced with stressful circumstances. I do not believe that SES is the major determinant of psychological resources available to handle threat.

Rather, what heart patients of all SES have in common is repeated exposure to invalidating experiences in childhood. There is scientific evidence quoted throughout this book, associating childhood invalidation with adult heart disease. Invalidation leads to shame and self doubt. Shame and self doubt deplete resources needed for dealing with threat or exercising self control. A heart patient with depleted reserves has less ability to delay gratification and curb impulses. He is more likely to engage in behaviors that worsen his heart condition.

Appendix A

RESEARCH ON CORONARY HEART DISEASE

The research presented here clearly implicates personality, behavioral, emotional and cognitive factors in the development and course of heart disease. These findings were published in The American Psychologist.

HOW CORONARY HEART DISEASE (CHD) DEVELOPS

CHD is typically first diagnosed in men in their fifties and women in their sixties, with men tending to present initially with a heart attack and women with angina or chest pain. These events are based on having plaque buildup that blocks sufficient flow to the heart muscle.

The buildup of plaque occurs over many years, and is thought to arise from the combination of endothelial dysfunction and inflammation. The endothelium is a layer of cells that lines the blood vessel. Dysfunction refers to the inability of the endothelium to inhibit platelet formation because of inflammation. Inflammation has been linked to lifestyle issues such as smoking, socioeconomic status, environmental stress, physical inactivity and non-compliance with treatment recommendations. Psychosocial factors play a role in damaging the endothelium, promoting and sustaining inflammation, facilitating adhesion of plaque to the arterial wall, and contributing to plaque rupture.

THE PSYCHOSOCIAL PREDICTORS OF CORONARY EVENTS

Research has focused on whether psychosocial characteristics predict who is at risk for coronary events among healthy participants or at risk for recurrent events among coronary patients. Stressful environments have been a primary target of research. Individuals working in jobs with high demands for performance and low decision latitude or jobs with high effort and low rewards have been shown to be at elevated risk for CHD events. Marital distress and poor communication were related to future events in CHD patients. With respect to personality characteristics, hostility, depression and anxiety have all been associated with coronary events.

THE PSYCHOSOCIAL PREDICTORS OF ATHEROSCLEROSIS

Several studies show that the lower the socioeconomic status (SES) the greater the aortic calcification and plaque. Similar results occurred with women dissatisfied with their marriages, and men in high stress jobs. Calcium and plaque buildup were significantly associated with measures of hostility and anger expression. Untreated hypertensive men who experienced anger frequently and expressed it outwardly had heightened carotid artery thickness, as did women who held their anger in. Anxiety, hopelessness, pessimism, and depression were also related to arterial calcification and plaque. These emotional states are natural consequences of repetitive invalidating experiences, in my opinion.

THE PSYCHOSOCIAL PREDICTORS OF ENDOTHELIAL DYSFUNCTION AND INFLAMMATION

It is known that a healthy artery dilates substantially in response to increased blood flow, while a diseased artery does not. One study reported that healthy women with higher anxiety and anger-in (experienced, but not expressed) scores had less dilation than women with lower scores. Higher scores on Type A behavior (competitive, impatient), anger and depression were also associated with less dilation.

A larger literature has examined the association of psychosocial factors with markers of coagulation and inflammation measured in the blood, such as C-reactive protein. Job stress, low SES, major depression, anger and anxiety have all been associated with inflammatory factors.

WHEN PSYCHOLOGICAL VULNERABILITIES TO HEART DISEASE BECOME EVIDENT

Early childhood socioeconomic status (SES) predicts the incidence of CHD in adulthood. Risk factors for heart disease, including obesity, high blood pressure, elevated lipids, cardiovascular reactivity to acute psychological stress, and hostility, track across childhood and adolescence and into adulthood. Obesity, high blood pressure and high levels of lipids in adolescents and adults predict coronary calcification, carotid thickness, and coronary atherosclerosis later in life.

From the above research we can conclude that psychological, environmental, and genetic factors all play a part in the development of heart disease. Obviously you cannot do anything about your genetic make up. But your genes are only part of the picture. Genes may predispose you to having a heart condition. In the majority of cases however, whether or not you become a victim of heart disease is determined by your life experiences and lifestyle choices. You can gain control over your lifestyle by becoming more aware of the obstacles outlined in this book, and following the pathways around the obstacles.

Appendix B

MENTAL FLOSS

*(What follows employs a bit of poetic license.
I can't resist a good analogy.)*

From a physiological standpoint, heart health is very much dependent upon two aspects of the artery: its elasticity and openness. The more flexible the artery, the better able it is to relax and tighten in response to the body's demands. The more open the artery, the greater the blood flow. The more plaque, the more the blood flow is restricted. It is understood that plaque forms in response to an injury to the artery wall. Harmful dietary and environmental factors can cause such an injury. The injury elicits an inflammatory response. Part of this response includes platelet aggregation around the injury. These sticky cells accumulate in the damaged area and become plaque.

Consider that there is an analogous process occurring at the psychological level. Picture the mind as an artery. Flowing through the mind is information. Like the artery, the mind functions best when it is flexible and open.

The mind compares new information with stored information assumed to be true (beliefs). A flexible mind can adjust beliefs to accommodate new information. A rigid mind establishes defense mechanisms in order to maintain its faulty beliefs. Psychological defenses filter and restrict the flow of information.

Invalidating experiences are perceived by the mind as threatening. They injure the mind the way harmful dietary or environmental factors damage the walls of the artery. Just as plaque forms to repair an injury to the artery wall, defense mechanisms arise to protect the mind from perceived insults. The injury to the artery wall elicits an inflammatory response. The insult to the mind elicits inflammatory emotions. Just as platelets accumulate at the source of the injury to the artery wall, defenses are found wherever invalidation occurs. Just as plaque restricts blood flow through the arteries, inflammatory emotions inhibit the mind from processing information.

You need a process to open your mind and rid yourself of faulty beliefs- a kind of mental floss.

Appendix C

THE CORONATION OF KING LARRY
(HOW I DISCOVERED THE ROYAL VOICE)

Many heart patients present themselves as tough, strong, self confident and in control. We see and understand how arrogance is often the flip side of shame. That is, we cover up our fear of being exposed as inadequate by displays of arrogance and one-upsmanship. Other heart patients may appear shy and bashful on the surface. They too felt shame and feelings of inadequacy. However they compensate for felt deficiencies by trying to please people.

I opened the Center for Cardiac Wellness at about the same time that I began working as a corporate consultant. The differences in the two groups of clients awakened me to the fact that heart patients were "tough" customers. Coaching executives in the area of Leadership led me to learn a great deal more about the field of Emotional Intelligence. My corporate executives seemed to thrive under the intensive program, which sought to increase their emotional literacy.

What I found, to my pleasure, was that these leaders, many of whom were already successful in Fortune 500 companies, had an intense desire to learn about themselves, and could apply their enormous intelligence to this process. At the end of the 48 hour program, many corporate leaders opted to continue with me in "graduate school." I also learned that there was a big difference between my teaching the concepts of emotional intelligence to executives, and my living in a manner whereby I actually practiced what I preached.

When I began seeing cardiac patients, at about the same time as I started coaching corporate leaders, I found my experience to be very different. After about three sessions, I began to hear rumblings of dissatisfaction from my heart patients. One of my heart patients asked a question which seemed to typify how others felt as well. "I really haven't changed very much after the three hours, how much longer do you think I will have to come?" Even though these individuals started my program with the same enthusiasm the corporate executives had showed, and with the added incentive that their very lives were at stake if they didn't change, these patients lasted about ten hours on average before they unilaterally terminated treatment (as opposed to more than forty eight hours with my corporate clients).

One day I asked one of my more resistant heart patients why he felt therapy would not work. He drew a breath and said in all seriousness, "Don't you think that therapy and counseling is nonsense?" What did he think I would say? "You know, you are absolutely right. I have spent the past thirty years trying to con and deceive people into coming in for help even though they didn't need it. It was a great way for me to make a quick buck." What kind of person did he take me for? How suspicious he must have been, and how fearful of being conned he must have felt. Didn't he realize that his question would cut me to the core? Yet believe it or not, I would have asked the same question if the situation were reversed.

It turns out that other professional people have also observed that it was tough going when treating heart patients. Did you know that a woman with breast cancer is 40 times more likely to attend a support group than a woman with heart disease? You already know that 90% of patients who have coronary bypasses don't sustain changes in their unhealthy lifestyles that worsen their severe heart disease and greatly threaten their lives. Did you know that two thirds of patients who were prescribed statin drugs to reduce cholesterol stop taking those drugs within one year?

What makes heart patients so non-compliant is related to an inability to handle painful emotions. Painful emotions often break through defenses and add to the stresses heart patients experience trying to cope with heart disease. The stresses become overwhelming and deplete energy needed for self control.

Although I exercised regularly, I continued to eat the wrong foods. I pretended to myself that the one medication I took to lower my cholesterol and the other medication I took to keep my blood pressure from going through the roof, somehow would allow me to eat whatever I wanted. I rationalized that these medications were canceling out the bad effects of a high fat, high carbohydrate diet. The "normal" rules didn't apply to me; a "king" is immune. I was not subject to the usual consequences that mere mortals faced.

Based upon my personal and professional experience, many of the characteristics mentioned above can be thought of as manifestations of excessive preoccupation with the self. Such preoccupation often occurs in response to traumatic shaming and invalidating conditions in childhood. The personality constellation that develops to defend against difficult childhood experiences is often compensatory in nature. In other words, the person attempts to compensate for feelings of worthlessness, either by assuming an air of superiority or one of exaggerated kindness.

THE KING AND QUEEN

I was a good example of the type personality, which I refer to as "The King". ("The Queen" is my female counterpart.) I walked and talked in a haughty manner, behaved as if I were entitled to special treatment, appeared self confident and in control, demanded that things go my way, became impatient and irritated by the "incompetence" of others, required immediate gratification, and believed that the normal rules (applicable to most human beings) did not apply to me. On the surface, I was a showcase of strength. People reported that they were intimated until they got to know me.

Several of my heart patients presented the same picture. Sam had a long list of requirements for his wife and children. The list included having dinner ready at a specific time, having the leftovers treated in specific ways, the refrigerator arranged in a manner that made sense to Sam. If any of these requirements were not met, Sam would feel that he was not respected, and fly into a rage. Sam was proud of his exacting standards, and was not shy about voicing his opinions (although Sam preferred to regard his opinions as "facts").

"PRETENDERS TO THE THRONE"

Some of my heart patients would be embarrassed and ashamed to stick out in any obvious way. In fact, they would be astounded to be thought of as a king or queen. These heart patients prefer to be seen as deferential, unassertive, and bashful, just the opposite of arrogant. Yet upon closer look, many of these heart patients have similar characteristics to Sam and me. For example, I have observed that these seemingly shy types actually have the same degree of toughness or stubbornness. They too seem preoccupied with the self, strive for recognition, are sensitive as to how others react, and entertain fantasies of greatness. But they would be less likely to boast, and may react with self contempt or depression to perceived failure or criticism, rather than the overt displays of anger that Sam or I might display. They may be imperious, but it would be covered with a veneer of gentility.

Mary and Edith were two of my heart patients who I would classify as the more introverted types of "royalty". These women were giving to a fault. They never forgot a birthday. They gave of themselves tirelessly. Both took great pride in the considerable accolades and awards that were bestowed upon them for their work, yet they were shy and sensitive about receiving too much attention. Try to cross either of these seemingly bashful women, however, and you would have hell to pay. Insurance companies that didn't pay their bills or doctors who were not on the ball would attest that these ladies were tough as nails underneath their gentle appearances. These were two of my toughest patients. Appearing unassuming and deferential, their insightful and to the point questions or comments were delivered with the power of a knockout blow I didn't see coming.

Arthur is another of my heart patients who appears to be more of a quiet and humble type of king. Known as a person with great tact and diplomacy, Arthur nevertheless has lived life on his own terms. He had married and divorced frequently, started many business ventures that failed, had been estranged from his children, and was filled with remorse. Yet Arthur continues to have ambitious plans that border on grandiose, is stubborn, opinionated, and tough minded underneath his shy demeanor. Arthur has been both my strongest critic and my most ardent supporter.

DEVELOPMENT OF "ROYAL" BEHAVIORS

To clarify the above, it may help to see the development of "royal" behaviors in the following way: First, invalidating experiences leave the future heart patient feeling deficient, deprived and ashamed. Second, compensatory and defensive actions are taken to defend against these feelings by adopting an arrogant posture as Sam and I did. In some cases, a third step occurs. This happens when the arrogant behaviors are themselves punished. The person has to go underground with his or her imperious thoughts and behaviors, and adopts a posture of meekness and gentility as Mary, Edith and Arthur did.

It was not difficult for me to recognize and accept that I was an arrogant person. I used to joke about my need to be first at the buffet line, as did others who teased me about my kingly nature. In a somewhat playful manner, I used to hold out my hand for people to kiss, whenever I was feeling particularly proud of myself. I reasoned it was OK for me to be this way, because I could justify my "superiority" by my numerous accomplishments.

I was ashamed of my envy and jealousy. I had successfully buried all recognition of this emotion. I was only aware of my competitiveness and only a little puzzled by my continuous efforts to find fault with those I secretly envied. For example, I could never understand how my partner was able to relate to our professional colleagues in such as friendly manner. He would ask them about their work, marvel at their newest publications or awards. I was always polite with these same people, but secretly wanted to cut their heads off. I saw them as rivals, and was threatened by their successes.

Few heart patients will admit to being envious or needy. No self respecting king could find himself to be in a one-down position to any mere mortal. This is particularly true for Harry, one of my heart patients who would be categorized as a humble type of king. Harry took quiet pride in being a captain in industry, a philanthropist, a teacher and a mentor. He was always thoughtful and giving – would bring me an extra bottle of cold water on hot days. Harry appeared in the sessions to be serious and unhappy, yet he was unaware of this. He was starved for appreciation, nurturance and support but could not see this in himself.

In Harry's family of origin, there was no tolerance whatsoever for the expression of feelings of deprivation, or envy. Harry would have buried these painful feelings a foot or two deeper than a more arrogant type of king, such as me. Remember, the shy or quiet king became that way because his arrogant and overtly angry behaviors were totally unacceptable to his caretakers.

In the pursuit of peace of mind, and in a frantic effort to alleviate his feelings of deprivation and deficiency, the heart patient may attempt impulsive and reckless behaviors. For example, he may go on an eating binge, or make expensive purchases on a whim. While these behaviors may be attempts by the heart patient to fill a sense of emptiness, they never succeed.

These compensatory behaviors do not succeed because security does not depend upon having things. It depends upon handling things. The more you can handle, the better you feel about yourself. You can learn to handle your feelings of deprivation by re-thinking your situation. Is there anything you can learn from this situation? Is the situation really as desperate as you think? Can you break the situation down into parts, and handle one part at a time? "Do I really need something out there to make me feel better, or can I find something within myself to feel complete?"

Once I became aware of the royal self, I was in a better position to handle my painful experiences and the unhealthy behaviors they triggered. To live a healthy life, I had to abdicate the throne.

REFERENCES

Baumeister, R. (2008). How to boost your willpower. *New York Times, Nov 7*.

Eisenberg, L. (2006). *The number*. New York: Free Press.

Frankl, V. (1946). Man's search for meaning. New York: Pocket Books.

Goleman, D. (1995). *Emotional Intelligence*. New York: Bantam Books.

Jeffers, S. (1998). *Feel the fear and do it anyway*. New York: Ballantine Books.

Matthews, K. A. (2005). Psychological perspectives on the development of coronary heart disease. *American Psychologist, 60*, 783-796.

Miller, E. (2005). Change or die. *Fast company, 94* (May).

Ornish, D. (1990). *Dr. Dean Ornish's program for preventing heart disease*. New York: Random House.

Seibert, A. (1996). *The survivor personality*. New York: Perigee Trade.

Sweeny, S. (2008). *Transform stress into strength*. Enumclaw, WA: Annotation Press.

Tolle, E. (2005). *The new earth*. New York: Penguin Group.

Trimpey, J. (1996). *Rational recovery: The new cure for substance addiction*. New York: Pocket Books.

Van der Kolk, B. (1997). Posttraumatic stress disorder and memory. *Times, 14* (3).

Whitfield, C. L. (1998). Adverse childhood experiences and trauma. *American Journal of Preventive Medicine, 14* (4), 361-364.

CONTACT THE AUTHOR

You can contact the author by visiting Dr. Decker's website:

DrLawrenceDecker.com.

Tell your story. Connect with others. Read blogs and articles.

ABOUT THE AUTHOR

Lawrence A. Decker received a Ph.D. in Clinical Psychology from Brigham Young University in 1970 and was a Post Doctoral Fellow at the Menninger Foundation.

Dr. Decker is a member of the American Psychological Association and a Fellow of both the Pennsylvania Psychological Association and the Philadelphia Society of Clinical Psychologists, where he has led and served on numerous committees and is also a member of the New Jersey Psychological Association.

For the past 35 years he has been in the forefront of the movement to integrate mind and body. Dr. Decker helped establish and direct The Achievement and Guidance Centers of America (AGCA), a managed healthcare company which merged into American Biodyne before being sold to Medco-Merck.

Dr. Decker is the director and founder of the Center for Cardiac Wellness. He continues to counsel patients in his private practice.

In conjunction with U.S. Healthcare, now Aetna , Dr. Decker helped develop and pilot a unique program integrating traditional mental health services into primary physician offices. Dr. Decker served on the Professional Standards and Review Committee for U.S. Healthcare, which later became Aetna. As a consultant to U.S. Healthcare, Dr. Decker trained psychologists to interface directly with physicians in the specific treatment of heart disease and other chronic diseases.

For the past eight years he has trained key corporate executives to become great leaders in companies such as McDonalds, Sovereign Bank, Penske, and American National Power. He continues to teach executives how to become more emotionally intelligent.

Dr. Decker is on the staff at Doylestown Hospital where he develops and delivers lectures and workshops for heart patients and medical personnel.

Dr. Decker is the author of a book, *A Change of Heart*, published by Nova Science Publishers in 1998.

Dr. Decker has been married to his wife, Louise, for the past 23 years. They live near the ocean and love to take walks on the boardwalk. Their son, Jay, is 17 and is obsessed with football. Dr. Decker has a daughter, Elena, a free-lance writer and illustrator, who lives in Georgia with her amazing husband and two handsome grandkids. Dr. Decker loves tennis, cross country skiing and is "starting to enjoy" golf.